# YOU NEED HUMOUR WITH A TUMOUR!

# YOU NEED HUMOUR WITH A TUMOUR!

# REFLECTIONS ON A JOURNEY WITH CANCER

**ANNMARIE JAMES-THOMAS**
**with JEREMY FLYE**

Published by Accent Press Ltd – 2013

ISBN 9781909624665

Printed and bound in the UK

To Geraint – my husband, my rock, my everything.
I'd never have finished this book without you.

# Foreword

*Tracey Burke, manager of Cancer Aid
Merthyr Tydfil*

I can remember the first meeting I had with Annmarie James-Thomas as if it were yesterday. It started with a typical telephone call from our reception volunteer to let me know that a new patient had arrived in the drop-in centre. I went down to meet Annmarie and her (as I would soon discover) ever-present husband, Geraint, and led them to the meeting room where all our new referrals are taken. I went through the usual procedure of taking her details and explaining the range of services that we provide, not just for her but for any family member. Then I listened as Annmarie voiced her concerns about her diagnosis, and we discussed what services she might require from us.

But hearing Annmarie talk was extraordinary because, in all the years that I have been working in this field, I have never before come across anyone who originally refused treatment from the onset after a cancer diagnosis. I kept looking from Annmarie to Geraint and thinking to myself: "This is a young woman with a family who is refusing treatment. This woman is absolutely crackers – what is she thinking?"

We sat and chatted for hours and I explored all the avenues with her – the who, what, when, where, how and why, if you like – as we discussed all of the issues surrounding her diagnosis. But it quickly became apparent to me, as it is to everyone that knows her, that Annmarie was a very strong and determined woman, and nothing anyone said to her was going to change her mind.

Over the weeks, and then months, that I got to know Annmarie, when she and Geraint came in to use the complementary therapies that we provide, one thing struck me: she always remained positive throughout. Never one to complain, she would always find something to laugh about. Yes, of course there were one or two occasions where it was emotional; sometimes when Annmarie was particularly poorly, and she couldn't attend the session that was booked for her, the girls and I would just look at each other. No words needed to be said: we were concerned that Annmarie was deteriorating and one of us would ring Geraint to see how she was. But it was almost as if our fears were groundless, for the next week she would be in to see us again, larger than life as always. She'd always make light of how ill she had been after treatment, and there was always a laugh and joke about how "it could have been worse, Trace – I could have had this side-effect or that side-effect". Every time, she has found and used the humour of her situation to get her through the side-effects of her treatment. You could see that Annmarie was one lady who was not going to let this illness get her down. What an inspirational woman!

We all make choices in life and, whenever we make a decision, whatever we decide is the right decision for us at that time. Later on, for whatever reason, we may question ourselves and think "maybe I should have done that differently" or "maybe I shouldn't have said that". Really, second-guessing yourself is pointless and a waste of time: we cannot change the past, but we can enjoy the present, and this is exactly what Annmarie has done every day of her life. And anyone reading this book will understand why those decisions were made at the time of her diagnosis.

When you've experienced the cancer journey, you change as a person; you appreciate all the small everyday things in life that we normally take for granted. Having support to see you through the tough times is a massive help to anyone, and having plenty of love and laughter in your life certainly goes a long way towards giving you a positive state of mind. That's Annmarie to a T. You will cry with laughter throughout this book, and you will cry with emotion for a young woman fighting an illness with such courage and determination.

There is always hope and new treatments are being developed all the time, but nothing can prepare you for the day when a clinician tells you that you have cancer – and then it is very much up to you as an individual to cope with the cancer journey. It's a lonely road and, no matter how much support and love you have from family and friends, you have to make the important decisions about which path to follow alone. There is no right or wrong way to deal with an illness of any sort; it is up to each individual to take whatever path feels right for them at that particular time in their life. This book is about an individual's cancer experience, the choices she made, and how she coped with a cancer diagnosis.

Annmarie made it work by having loving people around her who made her laugh. Read the book, and understand the woman.

# Being Thankful

How thankful am I – and is it enough?

I am so thankful for everything in my life – starting with me. I like the person I am. I am thankful that I am a spiritual person and that I am able to pass my knowledge on to others and hopefully help them on their journey of enlightenment.

I am thankful for my husband who is also on this journey. As one, you can achieve most things; as two, we can achieve anything! I love him with all my heart.

My children – how much they have enriched my life. I'm sure I would have been a different person without them. To be blessed with one child is truly amazing, but to be chosen by four of the most beautiful spirits is a miracle, and the best blessing anyone can hope for – I am honoured to know them. I love you so much.

My parents, my nan and my sister have indulged me in being the person I am, and I am truly thankful for their patience and support through the good and not-so-good times. Knowing you were always there has kept me moving forward. Thank you.

Friends – of whom I have many – I am thankful for. Good friends, I have very few of, and for these I am truly grateful. One of my greatest friends (I met her when I was 11 and I didn't know she would be that at the time!) – she knows who she is and I am so thankful for having her in my life and for all of her support. She is an amazing person.

This is how thankful I am just for the people in my life. I am thankful for so much more.

Is it enough? I truly don't know; I would hope it is. If it isn't, I wish for the inspiration to be more thankful and to live my life in gratitude.

# Chapter One

## I Always Knew I Was Going to Get Cancer

*Within everyday ordinary people, if you look closely,
you can find some extraordinary things*
**Joseph L Badaracco**

The comedian Spike Milligan once said that, when he died, he wanted to have the words "I told you I was ill" carved on his headstone. I'm the same, because I always knew I was going to get cancer. I know that sounds silly, or like I'm making it up now because I have it, but it isn't. I've always been spiritual – a bit psychic, if you like – and have often seen things "happening" to me before they do. And so there was always this feeling, a bit of a premonition really, that at some stage in my life I would get cancer.

It's not just me – my grandmother, Peggy, is very much the same way, though I think that it's a little more developed in her case than mine. And I think that it's this spiritualism and faith in God that has helped me deal with being diagnosed with cervical cancer, and given me the strength to follow my own path to conquering it.

Now don't get me wrong, I'm no one special: I'm just a typical 40-something housewife and mother of four from Merthyr Tydfil. At the time of the diagnosis I was living in a nice house on a nice little development on the outskirts of town with my husband

3

of more than 20 years, Geraint, our four boys – Zack, 22; Harrison, 18; Harvey, 16; and Roddy, now 13 – and our slightly smelly pooch, Lulu. We had the same stresses and strains as everyone else.

But fate chose to lob a dirty great stone into our little pond when, in April 2011, I was diagnosed with cancer of the cervix, following months of pain and medical investigations. And, since then, my life has been anything but typical, as I chose to meet my cancer head on. The last thing I wanted to be seen as was a victim. "Don't ever feel sorry for me" is what goes through my head all the time, because I'm not feeling sorry for myself.

Having watched my dad, Roy, succumb to bowel cancer almost two years before I was diagnosed, I had no desire to follow the same treatment regimen that he had undergone. Instead I went in search of something different. My journey since diagnosis has been literally that, taking me across the Atlantic in search of another way of combating the tumour that was growing slowly – then not so slowly – within me. The lessons I learned there about how to change the way I ate and drank, to effectively clean up my lifestyle and stop the cancer spreading, I've brought back home with me and tried to put into practice.

It's been hard, sometimes very hard. But there have been lots of highs along the way to counterbalance the lows. And that's why I want to tell people about what I did, and why I did it my way rather than the conventional way.

Soon after I decided to write this book, I talked about it to a friend. Strangely enough, he had just finished reading *Ripley's World*, an autobiographical look at international rugby player Andy Ripley's fight against prostate cancer. Despite coming from a family of rugby fanatics, I didn't know much about him – he was an English rugby player after all – and my friend told me that though Ripley had died in 2010 he had refused to be defined by his disease. But what my friend said about the way Ripley was first diagnosed with cancer was particularly interesting. Ripley had been admitted to hospital after suffering what was thought to be a heart attack. Tests revealed that it had actually been a pulmonary embolism, but blood tests showed an exceptionally high PSA (prostate specific antigen) reading – for a normal man of his age the reading should have been 3.5 nanograms per millilitre, but Ripley's was an incredible 135 ng/ml. But what really interested my friend was this: during his time in hospital Ripley came into contact with two distinct groups of patients – those with heart conditions and those with a variety of cancers – and was struck by the difference in the way in which the two groups acted after being diagnosed.

The heart patients, according to Ripley, were there because they were old, because they were stressed, because they had abused their bodies with drink, cigarettes or food (or a combination of the three), or it was genetic. But once they had come to terms with the fact that they weren't going to die – or at least not at once – they were a fundamentally happy bunch. The stereotype of the fat jolly man and woman seemed to be pretty much on the button, at least as far as Ripley was concerned. This was in stark contrast to the oncology wards and waiting rooms, where, Ripley wrote, "cancer, in its many forms and many stages gradually draws life out of the bodies of its victims. Not much happiness or quick death there, at best a gallows humour and a brave acceptance and resignation."

And when I thought about it later, I realised that Ripley had a point. Just look at the way we talk about cancer; no one even likes to use the word – we talk about "The Big C". And it's also true that people seem to become nothing more than their condition. They become less people in their own right than a collection of symptoms. Jeremy Flye, who helped me with this book, told me that his father, Derek, also had prostate cancer; he was diagnosed with it more than a decade ago and it was successfully treated, but then it returned in 2009 when his PSA count started to sky-rocket once more. Derek's life became a series of appointments and tests, injections and tablets. Holidays had to be fitted around injections, and if he missed taking a tablet he immediately started to worry. Check-ups became times of worry, for at least a fortnight before. If the PSA count went up, he was inconsolable; if it stayed the same, or went down, the immediate euphoria was followed by a post mortem ("Why do you think it went down? Is it something I did right this time?"). And though he carried on with his many sporting interests, Jeremy reckoned his dad's world became a lot smaller and he stopped finding joy in the small things.

Now I didn't want to do that. "Hi, I'm Annmarie. I'm an alcoholic" might be all right for Alcoholics Anonymous, but I'm not an alcoholic. I've got cancer, but it isn't who I am.

The other thing that Ripley highlighted was the loss of a sense of humour, not just in people who have cancer but those around them. And looking back on my experiences with people who have had cancer, as well as my own, I think that is very true. People tiptoe around you, it's almost as if they don't want to offend or say anything that can be taken the wrong way. Now everyone who knows me will tell you that I'm never short of something to say, and I'm never shy of offering an opinion when I'm asked (and sometimes when I'm not). And that was how I wanted people to be around me, and by and large I think I've succeeded in achieving that. The result is that I've managed to find lots of laughs in what some people would think of as a matter of life or death. There has been humour with my tumour. And I hope that will come out here.

# Chapter Two

## Dad is Diagnosed

We are not human beings having a spiritual
experience. We are spiritual beings having
a human experience.
*Pierre Teilhard de Chardin*

I didn't realise it at the time, but the first steps on my
journey to where we are today were taken in April
2007, four years before I was actually diagnosed,
because that was the time my dad was told he had
bowel cancer.

At the time of his diagnosis, Dad was only 57, but
he looked 20 years younger. He really did have a
passion for living – he was a larger-than-life character
who loved his food and drink – and so a diagnosis like
that was absolutely the last thing we expected to
happen. I know everyone says that but it really was
true.

The day the doctors told him, Mam phoned me in
hysterics just after they'd had the news. Dad hadn't
been too good for a few weeks, and they'd gone down
to the Royal Glamorgan Hospital in Llantrisant for
tests a few weeks earlier, but we all thought it was just
a blockage and so we weren't too worried about the
results. And after all, they were booked to go on
holiday to America in a few weeks so everything was

bound to be OK. But when they went into the waiting room, Mam and Dad were greeted by the sight of a nurse wearing a name tag with the job title "Cancer Nurse" – and that was when the penny started to drop. And when it dropped, it really did hit the ground with a crash.

The doctor who talked them through the results explained that the tests had revealed a mass which would require major surgery to remove it. In all likelihood, the doctor said, my dad would need a colostomy and then, after the operation, courses of chemotherapy or radiotherapy. But, said the doc, they needed to act fast: "If you don't have the surgery now, you won't be here by Christmas."

This was too much for Dad and Mam to take in, yet they had to. Obviously things were really bad and the cancer was quite advanced – without the surgery, the doctors reckoned that Dad had a maximum of eight months. But while it sounds like a no-brainer – have the op straight away – it wasn't quite that clear-cut for my dad. He was a very proud man, very dignified – I think most men of that generation were – and very neat, tidy and fastidious in his appearance and personal grooming. So the idea of a colostomy was horrifying for him. I genuinely think he would sooner have died than suffer what he would have felt was the indignity of that.

When Mam and Dad came back, we were all very low obviously, but we realised that this was just one doctor's viewpoint and we wanted a second opinion. Then Geraint remembered that a friend of his father's had undergone a colostomy operation himself, so we got in touch to get some idea for my dad about what having the procedure would actually involve. But we also asked him which doctor he had seen and whether he would recommend him. He gave us a name; we rang the London Clinic in St Mark's Hospital on the Monday, and on Wednesday Mam and Dad were sitting in the consulting rooms of Professor John Northover M.A.

Like most surgeons, Professor Northover cut straight to the chase. "You don't need a colostomy, and we can fix this." His confidence certainly buoyed up Mam and Dad, all the more so when he told them that he could do the operation when they came back from the States and they wouldn't need to cancel their trip. And so the surgery was penned in the diary for June. We didn't know this at the time, but the Professor is one of the country's most eminent colorectal cancer surgeons and had written the Royal Society of Medicine's handbook for patients with bowel cancer. We definitely felt we had the right man for the job.

So, with some sense of optimism, Dad went up to London for his operation after the holiday. Professor Northover had told Dad that he would almost certainly be in hospital for 14–17 days' postoperative care. In the event Dad was only in for seven days before discharge because the operation went so well; and though the journey back to Wales by private ambulance – that was me with my ambulance driver's hat on – was horrendous, the recovery itself continued to go well and we thought everything was on the up and up. But when Dad went back to hospital for his check-up, the tests showed that the cancer had spread to his liver. So once again he went back for another cancer operation, only this time half his liver was removed. But Dad continued to recover well and once more we thought there were grounds for optimism. Certainly he seemed so much better in himself.

But when he went back for his next check-up they found the tumour had once again metastasized to the liver and to the lymph nodes as well. Bowel cancer really is a horrible form of cancer – it's not as if there are any good ones though – but once it enters the body, it can quickly spread to other organs, including the brain.

So the next step for Dad was chemotherapy, and he went through the whole range of treatments in a bid to keep the cancer under control. He was taking steroids so his face became puffy, and he lost hair because of the chemo, but he was still the same fastidious Dad. And we were still able to laugh even as things became more difficult.

One week Dad was going into a palliative care facility to visit his care team. Now, like most men of his age, he didn't really "do" clothes or fashion – Mam would put his clothes out for him each night, washed, pressed and ready; and all Dad had to do was slip them on the following morning after washing and shaving. He never questioned her choices – after all, she'd never got it wrong and this was how it had always been. But on this particular day, Mam had put out some summer gear, namely a pink shirt and cream trousers. He came downstairs dressed and said: "I'm just going to phone Annmarie." "Why's that?" said Mam. "What's wrong?" "Nothing, but I just want to tell her that you've dressed me up like a bastard gay!" he said. That was funny, but that was also the day that Dad really gave up the fight because that was the day that the doctors told him that the cancer had spread to his brain.

It was getting harder and harder for Dad but, even then, he kept on going and it was a big thing for him to go up and down the stairs. No matter how ill he felt, each day he would come down from the bedroom to spend his day, and then go back up to bed in the evenings. And he always did it under his own steam. And whenever you asked him how he was feeling, no matter how he really felt, the answer was always the same: "Marvellous, marvellous!" But then one day he fell while going down the stairs, and that was the day Mam and Dad decided that they had to get a stair-lift fitted in their house.

And then, God love him, he started to lose parts of his vision and he moved into the conservatory. But even then there were so many funny things. Like the time we were watching the BBC2 quiz programme *Eggheads* on the TV in the conservatory. Now *Eggheads* has a segment where one team member is shown behind his or her team mates on a big screen as he takes part in a head-to-head round. Dad took one look at the screen and said "My God, look at the size of that bloke. They've got a giant in that team!"

And from there he decided that he wanted to let go. First Dad asked his doctor if he would increase the dose of medication. The doctor naturally declined to do so, so Dad's next step was to refuse to take his medication, knowing that this would most definitely kill him. One day, he just got up and said: "I'm not taking it." And that was that. He stopped.

Now you can talk about palliative care, but I think my dad is the only man to get his palliative medication from Reims in France. Dad and Mam always liked a nice glass of wine, and the only thing they liked more than a nice glass of wine was a very nice glass of wine. And they both had a weakness for Champagne. And Geraint and I knew this, and we also knew that, while they'd had some good ones, the one they had never tried was Louis Roederer Cristal, the drink of footballers and rock stars. So we bought them a bottle and when we opened it they were thrilled. "It's very drinkable," said Dad. "The price they charge, it bloody should be," thought I. Then my sister Kath bought a few more cases, so they carried on drinking it. Dad drank it the day before he died in October 2009. On the day he passed on, we had just one bottle left – which is kind of apt really. So we opened it and toasted his memory. Then I started making the calls you always have to make on days like this, and at some stage my mother's priest from Merthyr, Father Michael St Clair, called to pay his condolences and discuss funeral service arrangements. Once the champagne had gone, we'd started on some wine, and when that was gone we gave Mam lemonade – she didn't even notice. But when the undertaker called to meet my mother and begin making the arrangements, we had to open the door because she was three sheets to the wind. There was no option but to be honest, so I told the undertaker: "I'm sorry, but you'll have to come back tomorrow. The priest is here and Mam is pissed!"

Mam and Father Michael were drawing up the plans for the funeral and trying to decide on an order of service, but she couldn't remember the name of one of Dad's favourite hymns – it was *How Great Though Art* – so she ended up singing and humming the tune to him at the top of her voice while under the influence of Champagne. Anyone walking in on that would never have believed it – but Dad wouldn't have wanted her, or us, to be any other way.

It was an honour to give the eulogy at Dad's funeral, as it not only gave me closure but also the chance to tell everyone how much that marvellous man had influenced us: It might be a bit self-indulgent to reproduce what I said then here, but it's my book so if you don't like it ...

*I am so proud to be standing here and able to talk about an amazing man, Roy, who I am honoured to call my father.*

*Mam, Kath and I always knew that he was special*

*and I would like to share a little story with you about a holiday Mam and Dad took to one of the Greek Islands, Rhodes. Dad would have a go at anything and fancied a go at hang-gliding. Mam was going to ride in the back of the boat that was going to launch Dad in the air and take pictures. Mam was in the boat while Dad was harnessed up with the parachute on and he had to run along the beach while the boat built up speed before launching him up – this was the norm. However, he was far from the norm!*

*He ran along the beach, but being a giant of a man the boat wasn't going fast enough to drag him up into the air quickly, so it was travelling further out to sea from the beach, so Dad kept on running – only now he was running on top of the water. So when you hear the story of Jesus walking on the water in future, you now know someone else who did it.*

*As a family we have been so blessed – and our faith has carried us through the good times and the not-so-good times, the happy and the sad times, and we are grateful for all of them. We shared them together and got through them together, and this will always be the case. Dad's broken, pained body has left us but his spirit and the love we feel from him is amazing and will be with us always.*

*There is one thing that we share today – that my dad, Roy James, touched all our lives in one way or another through the love and kindness he gave to others. There are our memories and we cannot lose them and no one can take them away. They are ours to keep and an example to live by. This was his legacy. Thank you, Dad.*

I think watching my dad go through his battle with cancer certainly gave me an insight to how to deal with long-term conditions. For almost 19 months all he knew was treatments and medications, and that was his daily routine. A few days before he died, Geraint asked Dad whether, if he had known what he was going to go through, he would have had all the treatment – the operation, the chemo – and Dad said "No". I asked him the same question later, and got the same reply, and this really upset me because I started thinking that while we had tried our best to tend to his medical and physical needs, we'd not looked at treating and healing his spirit.

I was brought up a Roman Catholic in Merthyr, and even though I don't see myself as particularly religious, I was baptised, confirmed and married in the Church. Geraint isn't a Catholic – though he's a Merthyr boy too, from a well-known local family – and our four boys all went to his old school, Cyfarthfa High School, rather than my Catholic one, Bishop Hedley. So as you can see, I'm not the most religious of souls. Even now, I still believe a lot of what we were taught about God at school and at church – I think that we were a bit brainwashed, looking back at it – and even though I have become more spiritual over the years, a lot of the Catholic doctrine is still in me and if anyone asked me what religion I was, I'd say "I'm a Catholic". Having said that, I think that my generation is less devout than those of days gone by, the people who'd try to go to Mass every day and would be in their seat at church every Sunday and on all the Holy Days of Obligation – those days that the Catholic Church considers to be particularly religiously significant.

My mother, Pauline, is a Catholic, but my dad was not, even though he was married in the Faith, and he was laid to rest in it too. But when he was diagnosed with cancer, I did think a lot about religion and going back to the Church, but for whatever reason it just didn't happen. Some of that might have been down to Dad himself, because he was never particularly religious – Mam was always the religious one, making sure we went to church and things like that, while his role was more one of supporting her in this – but he was one of the kindest people I have even known, a real gentleman and a true Christian. I can still remember a doctor telling us: "For all the hardship and pain you are going through, I've never seen such a happy home or family."

Certainly it made me think about what I might do if ever I was stricken with the same illness, and whether I would adopt the same approach as my dad or look for another way, I never expected that just 19 months later I would be faced with making just that choice. The second leg of my journey was about to begin.

# Chapter Three

## What's Wrong with Me?

I told you I was ill

*Spike Milligan*

It was around Christmas 2010 when I started to think I wasn't well, though Geraint says that he could tell something was wrong as I had been out of sorts for a bit longer than that. First of all, it wasn't anything you could put your finger on, or at least nothing that I couldn't easily – and, as it turned out, wrongly – explain away. I had started to have vaginal bleeding outside of the times when my period was due but, as my family have a history of vaginal problems – both my mam and nan had hysterectomies before they had turned 40 – I thought I was suffering from the early onset of the menopause as I was around that age too. There you are, job done: a simple explanation for what was wrong. No need to panic, nothing to see so let's move on.

But on New Year's Eve, things started to come to a bit of a head. We'd gone, as we do most years, to the Celtic Manor – a five-star hotel and golf resort (they staged the 2010 Ryder Cup there) on the outskirts of Newport – to see in the New Year and combine it with some golf for Geraint and the boys. I'd had a bad stomach all day, and didn't know if I was going to start my period. Anyway, I had something to eat and went to bed, still with an upset stomach.

The following morning Geraint and the boys got up to play golf. I arose in a more leisurely fashion and went to the toilet, but started to worry a bit when I saw massive clots of blood in the bowl. Obviously this was a bit more serious so I made an appointment and went to see my doctor at the Morlais Medical Practice in Merthyr. The doc took samples and prescribed a course of antibiotics just in case. But when there was no improvement over the course of a week, I went back. This time the doctor took more blood samples and urine and also arranged for me to have an ultrasound investigation and a CT scan on my bladder. (An MRI scan had not been recommended – and at the time I was glad about that because I am incredibly claustrophobic and the thought of going into that tunnel really turned my stomach. In hindsight, perhaps it would have been better if it had been, as it would have helped the doctors make a diagnosis faster. I think that early MRIs should be used to help detect conditions as soon as possible.)

The CT results came back and showed nothing – (if you can *show* something that isn't there!) – but I was still living in pain. No, I was now living in agony and I kept asking myself why. Geraint was getting more concerned too, because he could certainly see that the pain was bad, worse than anything that I, a 40-something woman with a high pain tolerance – I had given birth to four children, naturally and with no pain relief, not even an aspirin – had ever felt before. He wasn't shy about telling me he was worried either and, as he said, something had to be done.

So, rather than let things lie, I went to London and paid to have a CT scan done as a private patient. And yet this too showed nothing and gave me the all clear as far as my bladder was concerned. But now the pain was getting so bad I did something that I'd never done before – I went to my GP and got him to prescribe me painkillers, and he also booked me in to go to Prince Charles Hospital in Merthyr for a colposcopy examination, which is where they run a camera down into your bladder. When they put the camera in they could see what looked like a blockage or cyst. The next step was an appointment with specialist Urology surgeon David Jones at the Royal Glamorgan Hospital. He wanted me in at once for a biopsy on my bladder, and his words really did send a chill down my spine when he said: "It's lucky you didn't leave it any longer, otherwise you'd be dead." Leave it any longer? I'd been to-ing and fro-ing between doctors and hospitals for the last couple of months – it was now February – but I still did not know what might be wrong.

I went back in on Wednesday for a pre-op but the doctors said I was overweight (I was tipping the scale then at around 28st), my blood pressure was through the roof and the anaesthetist said it was too high to operate safely, so David Jones told me to lose weight and come back in three months. So home I went, but still in pain and still without a diagnosis. But people who know me well know that I don't tend to let things go by without giving them a bit of a helping hand, so I went on to the Internet and started doing some research. The Internet is a marvellous tool and it's amazing what you can find on it – a couple of clicks and I discovered that there was an open (not enclosing) MRI machine at the Wide Open Centre of Cardiff, based at Cardiff Gate, at a cost of £200 for the scan, a disk of the session to take away, and a report. We rang them and were told we couldn't just turn up – we needed a referral letter from our GP. We organised that and trundled down to have the scan on a Friday morning. But the staff said we couldn't have the scan – the GP referral letter had not been specific enough for their needs. I felt they were being difficult but for once I kept my temper – and my tongue – in check and we said, as nicely as we could: "We'll sort out the letter with the GP. But as we are here can we just have the scan now please?" When I came out after having the scan, the staff could not have been nicer – I think they saw how upset I'd been before and the tea and biscuits were flowing freely.

Everyone has heard of MRI scans and scanners, but I don't think many people know that much about them. "MRI" stands for "magnetic resonance imaging". This is a radiology technique that is used to visualise the body's internal structures in great detail. Basically, MRI uses something called "nuclear magnetic resonance" to make a picture of the atoms that comprise a human body. And, for most of us, that's as much science as we need to know. The MRI scanner which is used to take the picture is basically a large ring magnet that you lie in and which effectively spins a magnetic field around you and, by the wonders of technology, creates a three-dimensional picture of your body, with all its lumps, bumps and imperfections. And, unlike CT scans, it does not expose you to any radiation – CT scans use X-rays to form a picture. In my case, the 3-D image that the scan captured was then stored on a disk so that doctors could use it to diagnose what was causing so much pain.

On Monday April 4, I went back to my GP surgery to go over the report and disk. After all the long drawn-out procedures I wasn't expecting to hear anything concrete, and so I drove myself up; Geraint was at work and the kids were in school. Sitting in the waiting room, I made some small talk with other patients, and was soon called in to see one of the young female doctors at the practice. "Sit down," she said almost as soon as I walked through the door. "It's not good news, I'm afraid." I asked her to read out the letter, and as she read a few words and phrases seemed to jump out from the medical jargon – the key ones were "cancer", "Stage IIb", "cervix" and "5.5 centimetres".

Was I surprised? I don't know for sure – after all, I always knew I was going to get it at some stage in my life. So I suppose I took it pretty calmly. But the young doctor was terribly upset and was crying. So there we were, the professional who had just broken the news of a patient's cancer being comforted by the woman she'd just given the diagnosis to. Don't let anyone tell you that doctors don't care about their patients: my doctors at Morlais all care about their patients, very deeply.

So as I got back in the car, I started to think about what I'd just heard. That was it, the jury had returned. I had cancer of the cervix, the tumour was 5.5cm long and it was Stage IIb. Now this last bit – Stage IIb – needs a bit more explaining, because it was not something I'd really heard about until my dad was diagnosed. When cancer doctors and nurses talk about the stage of a cancer, they are basically talking about how far the cancer has spread in a patient. There are different stages in the development of a cancer, numbered progressively from I to IV – why they use Roman numerals instead of the good old 1,2,3,4 is beyond me, but there you go. There is also a stage before Stage I called, naturally enough, Stage 0. What stage you are diagnosed as having depends on a number of factors, like the size of a tumour, how far it may have penetrated into the wall of a hollow organ and whether it has spread to organs near the tumour. The staging gives you an idea of what chance a patient has of survival, and tends to dictate what cancer treatment is followed.

As a simple guide, Stage 0 is an early form of cancer where the cancer cells have not actually spread into the surrounding tissue. Stage I refers to cancers that are localised to just one part of the body, whereas Stage II and Stage III cancers are locally advanced. Whether a cancer is classified as Stage II or III sometimes depends on the specific type of cancer. In Stage IV, the cancers have often metastasised to other organs or moved through the body. Now in my case, the MRI indicated Stage IIb cervical cancer – this meant that the cancer had spread into the tissues next to the cervix but had not spread to nearby lymph nodes or any distant sites.

The medical lesson over, let's cut back to me sitting in the surgery car park thinking to myself: "I want – I need – to get my head around this. Do I tell Geraint? Yes, I am going to need his support. Do I – which is now going to be 'we' – tell anyone else? No, it'll only mean lots of explaining and crying and sympathy, and I don't want to be anyone's sob story. I don't want it and I don't need it." That was the practicalities of the moment sorted out, but I was thinking of other things too – not least all the to-ing and fro-ing and time waiting to get tests done and results back. Once I'd had the MRI, a diagnosis had come quickly, but what if I hadn't been able to have the MRI privately? What if I'd had to wait for the NHS wheels to turn? Geraint and I were able to pay for a scan – not everyone is – but we could not believe how cheap it was comparatively. And also I was sufficiently Internet-savvy so I'd been able to find an open MRI scanner to get over my claustrophobia – but again, not everyone is, certainly not older cancer sufferers.

With Geraint on board, I made another appointment

to see a GP, and this time I was seen by my regular doctor, practice head Professor Jonathan Richards. Before I even sat down he said: "Just what did you do to my young doctor? She was in tears after seeing you!!" Before I could say anything, he carried on: "She told me what had happened, but when I saw it was you who had been the patient I told her 'she's tough as old boots, she can handle it'." I said: "Gee thanks, Doc!" and he replied "Well, at least you handled it better than some would have." We started to talk about treatment options and I asked Professor Richards what he'd do if it were his wife who had been diagnosed, and he didn't hesitate. "I'd get her straight in," he said. At this stage though, with the memories of my father's cancer still in my mind, I was already thinking of the possibility of exploring alternative options, but I let him go ahead and book an appointment with a consultant oncologist to confirm the MRI findings and review the medical options that were open to me.

Two weeks later I was sitting in the offices of Mr Rob Howells at University Hospital Llandough near Penarth. Rob is a gynaecologist and one of the senior members of the Cervical Cancer Team at Cardiff and Vale University Health Board, who duly confirmed that I did indeed have Stage IIb cervical cancer, and then outlined what treatment options were available to me. Surgery was not an option, he said, which left chemotherapy, radiotherapy or chemoradiation (a combination of the two). But I said "I'm not having it." When I told him I was looking at going down the route of a holistic, as well as just a medical, treatment, he was very supportive of my decision. I think he could see that I had been looking into the available treatments, and was not going to just accept that the only options were the medical ones. I'd seen my dad and his quality of life when he was undergoing conventional medical treatments: he was only having two or three good days a week, and that was when things were going well. There were alternatives out there, and I wasn't ruling anything in or out at this stage. So it made perfect sense to me when he said: "But I'd still like you to have a biopsy as soon as possible so we can see exactly what we are dealing with." After all, by doing this we were just covering every eventuality and amassing as much information as possible to help with my treatment. But I think my answer still shocked him.

"I can't," I said. "I've booked my flight and I'm going to America!"

Hats off to Rob Howells, he quickly got over the shock when I told him I'd decided to go there for a non-medical treatment and then outlined what I was going to try. "I'll support you all the way," he said, making it clear that the door was always open for me to come back and go down the medical route. We agreed that I'd go to the US and try the treatment there, and then come back for a scan in four months – and on that basis we arranged another appointment for August.

Having spoken to the oncologist, the next step seemed to be obvious: I had to tell my mother and sister. So, we rang them in the car on the way back from Llandough. Obviously this isn't the sort of thing you can tell someone over the phone; nor the sort of thing you want to have to say more than once if you can possibly help it. So we told Mam we would be coming to see her, and then rang my sister and told her to meet us at Mam's house. When we told them, my sister was quite hysterical while Mam was quite brave but once that moment had passed, my sister was on one laptop and her husband Steve was on the other, with all three of them looking at cervical cancer sites, to get information about the condition, potential courses of treatment and things like that.

It was difficult for them, I know, but I still tried to get my point over to them about the fact that I was looking at holistic therapies as well as conventional treatment. I told them that, if you look at cervical cancer websites, they will tell you that most cancer sufferers live another five to ten years after being treated for the condition. But I don't want to live for ten years at most – I want to be around for 30 or 40 years more than that and watch my children grow up and have children of their own, and then play grandmother to them. I don't know if I succeeded in convincing them at the time, but at least they knew what I was thinking.

The other person I had to tell was my best friend in the whole wide world, Avalon. We've been close ever since my mam started her shop in Merthyr, as Avalon was her first employee. But she's far more than that, both to me and to Mam. She had to know, because she's my sister – that's how I think of her. Even if she hadn't been my sister and my friend, I still would have told Avalon. I was worried that Mam would be unable to handle the pressure, and I'd want my best friend to know so she could keep an eye out to see that Mam was coping OK. So Avalon had to know: she was on the "people I have to tell" list three times over.

The boys were a different matter altogether. We decided that we wouldn't say anything to Zack, Harvey, Harrison or Roddy. After all, I truly believed that I was going to recover, and therefore the kids didn't need to know. I suppose that it's every parent's instinct to protect their kids, to shield them from bad news as much as possible, After all, Roddy was still in primary school, while Harvey was in Year 10 and preparing for some of his GCSEs and Harrison was in

Year 11 getting ready to complete his. We certainly didn't want to unsettle them. Zack was 20 but, as we weren't telling the others, there was no reason to tell him as he didn't have to watch out for their feelings or manage their expectations in any way. At home I was keeping things together, acting as if nothing was up – and on the surface that was true. Three of the boys didn't realise what was happening; but the exception was Harvey. Somehow he picked up that something was going on, but we played things down and he seemed to accept that.

Obviously though, with my preparing to be away for the best part of a month, we had to tell them something. Now, we had already explained some of my symptoms and hospital appointments away as "women's troubles" – that wonderful phrase that tends to have men heading in the opposite direction at 90 miles an hour as soon as they hear it (try it some time when you need to buy a new dress – it works wonders!) – so we said that I was going to do some courses and learn how to get over these "women's problems". They took the news pretty much in their stride – in fact, the thing that seemed to bother them most was that they were going to be subjected to the culinary skills of Chef Geraint Thomas who, as far as they knew, needed a recipe to make toast.

Apart from Avalon, none of my friends knew initially. Really my cancer diagnosis was on a need-to-know basis, and most people didn't need to know. Sometimes people ask me now why I didn't tell them sooner, and I say that I just didn't want them to worry about what they could do or say. That's true, but there was an element of selfishness in there too. Think about the way you behave with a friend or relative who has just announced that they have cancer or some other serious condition: when you hear the news the first instinct is to sympathise and try to make them feel better. I know; I've done it myself. People mean well, but the last thing I wanted or needed at that moment in time was a pity party – I just wanted to be myself and having people feel sorry for me would not help at all.

Actually, one person did know what was happening, and that was sort of forced on me by events. During the Easter holidays, just before I flew off to America we went to Weymouth as Harrison's rugby team was going on tour. I was trying to keep things as normal as possible during this time so that no one would pick up on the fact that I was unwell, or just how unwell I was. But Lauren Lewis, one of the coaches' wives, works in Boots the Chemist. She saw the amount of painkillers I was taking, realised that I was in some difficulty and asked me if I was OK. Well, I couldn't lie, so I told her what was wrong and asked her to keep it to herself as I wasn't telling anyone. Naturally she did, so that was good. After that some other of my closest friends were taken into my confidence, but very, very few.

Then, it was just a case of packing my bags and getting ready to be off. My flight was booked for April 30, which was Kath's birthday, and I'd be out in Florida for 21 days to undertake what was called a "three-week health encounter". Geraint drove me up to Heathrow – no one else came – and off I went: an afternoon flight to Miami, travelling First Class with Virgin Atlantic (remind me to tell Mr Branson that I think he's doing a great job).

And the next stop: Hippocrates.

# Chapter Four

## First Do No Harm

There's more than one way to skin a cat
***Proverb***

As my car drove me down from Miami International Airport to West Palm Beach on a late April afternoon, I was many miles away from Merthyr, both geographically and culturally, and I was counting on the change to do me good. But as we pulled onto the 40-acre estate that comprises the Hippocrates Health Institute, it really did feel like I was entering another world, with the tropical vegetation providing the perfect backdrop to my escape from external pressures. I could not think of a better place to learn about a way of eating myself back to health.

As we drove through the facility, it was hard not to look on it as if it were some resort hotel, and a pretty swish one at that. The accommodation ranged from two- and three-bed, two-storey villa suites, through to a hacienda-style building (which I discovered the next day was pretty much in the centre of the campus, near the lecture halls, spa and juice bar) and several luxury homes of varying sizes to accommodate families or groups of friends. The facilities too were impressive, and pretty much what you'd expect in a top-drawer spa hotel, including an ozonated recreational pool sauna, ozonated whirlpool and ozonated (yes, they are really

28

into ozonated water!) sea salt pools, a fully-equipped gym, and complementary electromagnetic therapies, spa and therapy treatments. And even though the scale was quite impressive, I pretty much knew what to expect, because, before choosing Hippocrates, I'd gone into things pretty thoroughly, and I knew what I was getting into.

Now reading this may surprise a lot of my friends, because I know that many of them think that when I decided to travel to Florida to learn how to change my lifestyle, I was effectively turning my back on traditional medicine and trying what some people might call "that holistic medicine crap". But that really couldn't be further from the truth. Of course I didn't give up on medicine – after all, while I was trying to be diagnosed – and after that too – I was being prescribed painkillers. And I suppose that this is something I would like to set straight. It wasn't a case of "either/or" – it was more "as well as". Once I started to take painkillers, and this was before I was diagnosed, I was taking the standard paracetamol-ibuprofen cocktail that will normally knock out an elephant. Then, when that didn't seem to touch the pain, I was prescribed Oramorph – but I didn't take it.

Nor was this some sort of cranky whim that I went off on: far from it. As soon as I was diagnosed, I went into Yahoo!- and Google-mode on my computer, searching out possible alternatives to the medical regimen that had ultimately failed my father. I had already come to think that his treatment had concentrated too much on the body at the expense of the spirit, and I think that you have to nourish and heal both.

All the information I could gather about alternative therapies suggested there were two main schools of thought: one is where you modify your diet to fight the cancer, while the other is more drug-based. For a variety of reasons, it was the diet-based therapies that most appealed to me, and as I searched on the Internet, one name kept coming back to catch my eye: Hippocrates.

Whoever came up with the name for the Hippocrates Health Institute, they did an excellent marketing job – it just reeks of medicine. And for me, it immediately conjured up the phrase "First do no harm" which is one of the principles of medical ethics, and which itself appears to be derived from the Hippocratic Oath. Nor is it offering courses of quack medicine treatments; set up in 2000 by Ann Wigmore, it is now run by a husband and wife team, Brian and Anna Maria Clement, both of whom hold a Ph.D.

Ann Wigmore is a particularly interesting lady who, back in the 1960s, founded a concept which she claimed was based on the principles of Hippocrates, namely "Let food be thy medicine". Along with Viktoras Kulvinskas, she set up an institute in Boston, Massachusetts, that "taught people how to access the power of their vast inner resources to transform the quality of their lives". The Clements have continued Wigmore's work at the Hippocrates Institute. Times have changed and there has been international recognition of the benefits of wheatgrass, which has coincided with the advent of natural approaches to healthcare. Modern research has identified direct links between certain foods and health risks, and Hippocrates is helping to educate people about disease prevention and the effects of positive diet and lifestyle choices.

According to the institute's website: "The Hippocrates philosophy is dedicated to the belief that a pure enzyme-rich diet, complimented by positive thinking and non-invasive therapies, are essential elements on the path to optimum health." The Clements help people radically change their health by teaching them how to trade what they term "nutrient-deficient, 'dead' foods" for something completely different: a diet rich in antioxidants, vitamins, minerals and plant-based proteins. The Hippocrates plan, which makes liberal use of fresh sprout and vegetable juices, wheatgrass, salads, nuts, seeds and fruit, supplies the oxygen, enzymes, alkalinity and bioelectrical charges which the Hippocrates Health Institute reckons are vital to cellular and general health.

Wigmore's own experiences seemed to back this up, according to the research I did. She came to America from Lithuania, and her family had a background in medicine. Her mother was a village doctor and Wigmore recalled her treating soldiers with herbs during World War I. She used many of these herbals remedies and techniques to treat and cure herself of colon cancer. Subsequently, Wigmore developed a way of life that she claimed provided "optimal health" for all its followers, based largely on the consumption of wheatgrass juice and a range of other vitamin- and enzyme-rich raw foods, and, according to the Hippocrates website, her name "is now synonymous with the history of the natural health movement that has pushed complementary healthcare measures to the forefront of US and world consciousness".

When I had told my family exactly what I was going to be doing at Hippocrates, the reactions were mixed. My sister Kath and brother-in-law Steve were not that keen at all. Geraint was on board, of course – we'd talked it all through beforehand – and Mam was all for it: "This is the way forward," was how she put it. And of course, she was right. Because of the stage my cancer was at, they couldn't operate – the only option was to shrink the tumour

I had booked to be at Hippocrates for three weeks and it was a time of swinging emotions for me. I laughed every day, and cried a lot too. Don't get me wrong: I'd chosen to go here but it would be wrong to pretend it wasn't hard too – I was homesick every day (this was the longest I'd ever been away from my family since Geraint and I had got together more than two decades before), I was in a hell of a lot of pain and I was on my own – no wonder I felt a bit isolated to begin with. Added to that, I wasn't eating. My appetite was completely shot.

Now food has always been a big part of my life. I've always eaten well and healthily, and if I say so myself I'm a good cook – but don't just take it from me: Geraint and the boys would be only too happy to give me a reference for my skills in the kitchen. I'd always been a healthy girl, a little more than average height compared to my friends, and a healthy weight. But over the years, eating well, though wisely, combined with a less active lifestyle, the demands of cooking for four growing boys and then eating with them meant that I started to gain weight. Though it was slow and imperceptible to begin with my weight crept up over the years. At my heaviest, shortly before I began to feel ill, I was 28st, though in the months after my diagnosis I lost a couple of stone. When I left for Florida I weighed 26st. But now, it was like I was brainwashed so I couldn't eat – the thought of food did nothing for me at all. Just the smell of food could make me feel ill. As I discovered, one of the side effects of cancer is this heightened awareness of aromas and smells, and it was the thing that made the early days so difficult. At the time of my diagnosis, they told me that some senses might become impaired but others might be heightened, and so it proved as my aversion to food seemed to come from the smell.

Even so, being off your food might not sound too drastic or even bad news on the face of it – after all, losing weight would make me healthier, right? And it's not like I didn't have weight to lose. But, and this is a big but, the whole point of the Hippocrates way to health is that you eat yourself well – it's by modifying your diet that you become healthy. And because I couldn't eat the food I couldn't modify my body chemistry.

To make sense of this, I'll take time out from my tale to tell you about the Hippocrates programme. To understand what I was going through you need to know a little more about the Hippocrates way and how, for it to work properly and effectively, it relied on my being able to eat the "right" sorts of food.

When I went to America, it wasn't to get cured, or at least not in a "take three pills twice a day and come back in a month" sort of way. It was all about learning how to change my lifestyle, and the three-week residential course was designed to teach us about the food that we'd need to eat in order to cleanse our bodies. In the lessons and seminars, the instructors looked at topics like detoxification, stress management, and a host of others, the object of which was to help us learn to make the body operate more effectively. The core of the message that the Clements and their instructors taught was the concept that the human body was pretty much like an alkaline battery.

Trying to make sense of this was a little daunting at first. I'm by no means dull – I defy anyone to say that of any woman who runs a family home – and since leaving school I have run a business successfully over a period of years, but I did leave school at 16. However, it was a lot like going back to Bishop Hedley

High and my physics lessons on magnetism and electricity, but a lot of what they said struck a chord – I must have been a better student than I thought, or there was more trapped in my subconscious than I realised. Basically, according to Hippocrates, each cell acts like its own battery, with a positive pole – the cell nucleus – and the negative pole – the cytoplasm. As the positive and negative charges collect at each pole of the battery, or the body, the potential for energy flow in a cell increases. And the greater the flow of energy, the healthier the cell becomes.

The body chemistry helps create these positive and negative charges. Some minerals are positively charged – acidic minerals – while others are negatively charged – alkaline minerals. And as carbohydrates are burned to release energy, these minerals are released into the body and acidic waste by-products are formed. And, according to the Hippocrates approach, to neutralise and eliminate these acidic wastes, the body need to have built up – and keep building – a store of alkaline reserves, a bit like savings in a bank that you can draw on in times of need.

Healthy cells have adequate reserves of alkaline and acidic charges in the cell, and a natural diet and lifestyle will help top up the necessary bioactive alkaline and acidic elements: this will then produce the maximum cellular energy and minimise acid waste products. So, in unhealthy cells there are inadequate reserves of bioactive acids, and probably too high a level of acid waste products that have built up over time: it's a two-stage thing. As a result, the charge between the nucleus and cytoplasm decreases in these unhealthy cells and the level of cellular energy resources drops; this in turn leads to the build-up of more metabolic acids, and the cycle repeats itself, leading to illness and disease. When the chemistry of the cells' cytoplasm becomes too acidic, and the potential energy in the cells falls below a level where life functions in the cells can be supported, cells will die. For this reason, Hippocrates teaches that it is necessary to keep the body at the right pH level.

Now most of you will remember the pH scale from your days at school, just like I did. It's an easy way to measure the acidity and alkalinity of anything. For those of you with an interest in chemistry – and that's not me, by the way! – it works by comparing the number of hydroxyl-forming alkaline ions with the number of acid-forming hydrogen ions. The scale runs from the most acidic at 0 to the most alkaline at 14, with the midway point, 7, being what scientists would call a "neutral pH". Water is composed of one hydrogen and one hydroxyl ion, and therefore has a neutral pH of 7, and because our bodies are 80%-composed of water, the human body also has an average pH of around 7. But the important word there is "average" and each individual cell has its own pH. A slightly alkaline pH (in the range 7.1–7.45) in a cell's cytoplasm is the level for optimum cell health, but most "averagely healthy" people have a pH in the 6.5–6.8 range. As a person's health declines, so the pH falls until what can only be likened to a fire alarm combined with a sprinkler system kicks in and the body's survival metabolism begins to produce ammonia (with a pH of 9.45) and brings the cellular pH back above 7. However, body pH does not tell the whole story and is only one small indicator of health. For example, kidney problems can lead to misleading answers to tests as they distort body chemistry. Also urine and saliva chemistries can vary depending on the time of day, diet, stress levels and other factors.

Now where all this affected me and my cancer was in terms of cell pH. According to Hippocrates, as cell functions become overburdened and acid-forming toxins collect in the cytoplasm, pH levels fall and the cells' potential energy decreases. This in turn minimises the transfer of oxygen and nutrients between cells and impacts on the elimination of toxins in cells too. And when acid levels reach a critical point, the cells die – or they mutate and become cancerous. So the challenge is to maintain – or retain in my case – the alkalinity in the cytoplasm of my cells. However, a combination of diet, exercise and positive thinking would allow me to face these "health challenges" (as the staff at Hippocrates called them) successfully. As the manual we were given, when we started the "three-week health encounter", states: "The Hippocrates diet provides all the life-enhancing oxygen, enzymes and bioactive vitamins and minerals that you need while minimising the by-products of waste that burden the body. Among the excessive acid-forming elements that you should avoid are polluted air and water, most household electrical appliances, non-organically grown vegetables and fruits, all meat (including chicken and seafood), dairy products, cooked food, overeating and negative thought."

The Hippocrates approach is based on the body's need for a balance of alkaline-forming and acid-forming natural vegetarian food. From years of research and clinical findings, the Hippocrates diet proposes that we follow an 80/20 rule, or as it puts it: "To replenish and sustain your proper alkaline and acid reserves, eat 80% of your foods from the alkaline-forming list and 20% from the acid forming list." For many women who are used to following diets where certain types of food are banned, or only allowed on certain days, this probably sounds quite straightforward. Men may find it a little more confusing as they – especially ones from my generation and ones before – would not be as aware of food-combining.

Among the alkaline-forming foods that were recommended on the course were small grains like millet or amaranth; sprouts of small seeds, beans and most grains; leafy and root vegetables; vine-ripened fruits/vegetables such as cucumbers and tomatoes; rarer sea vegetables such as dulse, nori and wakame; fresh herbs; cayenne pepper; garlic and onions; tree-ripened fruits; fresh beans and sweet corn. Freshly-squeezed green vegetable juices, drunk on an empty stomach, was a special treat.

The acid-forming list of foods is shorter, but includes those items that tend to be found in more store-cupboards and recipes. It includes those fruits that are not alkaline-forming, such as blueberries, cranberries, plums or prunes; some grains that have been soaked for 8–12 hours such as buckwheat or rye; and dry beans that have been soaked for 12–16 hours. Most nuts are acid-forming, but those that were acceptable after being soaked for 12–24 hours included pecans, hazelnuts, walnuts, almonds, fresh coconut and pine nuts. Seeds like pumpkin or sunflower, soaked for 5–8 hours, or sesame seeds (soaked for 3 hours) would also be permitted.

The Hippocrates diet also outlined what I would call an "amber" list of foods that, while not banned outright, would not be recommended either. On this were some of the more normally eaten staples, such as large grains like barley, rice, oats and wheat. Coffee was also frowned upon, presumably because it contained caffeine (though tea was not, funnily enough), as were tobacco, vinegar and processed condiments like tomato sauce, mayonnaise and mustard.

Some foods are red flagged – and just like any diet

you may have looked at or tried yourself, the ones to avoid tend to be the ones you're most likely to enjoy! Meats, dairy products, wheat flour, eggs, salt, refined sugars, alcohol and tobacco are consumables to beware of in the Hippocrates diet: not only are they acid-forming but they also cause the build-up of excessive amounts of mucous in the body.

The Hippocrates diet also identifies activities that could help balance acidity and alkalinity, as well as foods. Alkaline-forming activities included exposure to moderate sunshine, rest, exposure to fresh air (ideally sea air), fasting, relaxation, listening to soothing music, moderate exercise and drinking adequate volumes of water. Emotional and mental states that help form alkalines include laughter and things that build up your sense of worth and value. Acid-forming activities include cooking and preparing foods, a lack of rest, a lack of oxygen, overeating (too much and too often), stress, noise, the wrong amount of exercise (too little or too much) and dehydration. Emotional and mental states that help form acids include anger, confusion and fear.

In a nutshell – or at least an alkaline-forming nutshell – that was the food regime I was meant to be following. And it was a big change. Before I became ill, and certainly before I went on the Hippocrates diet, I was eating everything: pasta, bread, meat with gravy, spicy food, Indian, Chinese – there was no type of cuisine that I didn't like. Not only that but I was something of a Diet Coke addict too. And then, when I came to Hippocrates, I gave it up just like that – it was like cold turkey (oh yes, and I liked eating cold turkey too!). Before the diet started, I went through a detox process, and apparently I had such a bad detox the staff at Hippocrates told me that was why I was probably feeling so sick. And eating was the last thing on my mind right then.

So there I was – out in Florida, homesick, in pain, emotional, and unable to eat the raw-food vegetarian diet I was meant to be following. So I wasn't: I just could not hack it. I was staying in a place that resembled a five-star hotel in terms of facilities and ambience with excellent staff and all the support you could possibly ask for, but the food did not tempt me in the slightest. There were daily lectures and classes about diet, stress management, physiology and so on, as well as massages, spa treatments and time by the pool. And all that was great and totally absorbing. But the food? Oh no!

The staff were so worried about me to begin with, because I was so lethargic about the food on offer, that they even tried to excite me by cooking the food. A little sweet potato soup, to give me some nourishment at all, was the first thing they tried. After a couple of days of that when it seemed to go down OK, they moved on to the raw food diet: I started off with some lettuce and then some raw corn on the cob, which was so sweet it tasted like a dessert. However, I drew the line at dulse, a sea vegetable, a red alga which is apparently a seaweed that is much prized by the people of Iceland, Ireland and the north-eastern US. Well it was not popular with former pupils of Bishop Hedley High School, who thought it tasted rank! Full of protein, perhaps, but very unappetising (when I returned to Merthyr and looked at recipes using it, I wasn't surprised to see that many of them involved making it look – and taste – like something else). And another element of the Hippocrates diet that I never really warmed to involved raw garlic – or more specifically, eating two cloves of raw garlic. Every day. Every day? I mean, have you tried to eat one clove of raw garlic? What I would have given for some tiger prawns at that moment in time!

But worst of all was wheatgrass. By the end of three weeks, what I didn't know about wheatgrass preparation wasn't worth forgetting. But the most important thing I knew about wheatgrass was this: it made me puke. A lot. And often. And when I say "often" I mean "every time they tried to get me to take it". Everyone had to drink a portion of wheatgrass juice twice a day. The staff cut it fresh each day, and kept it in fridges near to the juice bar. But the smell of it turned my stomach, even though we were taking it like a sort of medicine. I couldn't stand the stuff, and I've got a strong stomach. So then, in desperation they tried to deliver it anally – they put it in a syringe and squirted it up my bottom. Now this was one they'd never believe on the Brecon Road! That night I phoned Geraint: "Guess what I did today? I let them put wheatgrass up my bum." Bless him, Geraint was horrified: "Bloody hell, Annmarie – those stalks are about 8 inches long!" When I stopped crying with laughter, I explained to my poor confused husband that they juiced the stalks before injecting them – so it was liquid that was going up my bum, not the grass stalks themselves. I think Ger was relieved as he had a mental image of me with a green bushy tail hanging out of my bottom. If he was embarrassed at my reaction, he would have been really shocked at the hysterical yelps from the other residents at Hippocrates when I told them.

As well as the treatments and therapies, everyone had a daily enema as part of the detox. That was fine, but they also offered everyone a complementary colonic irrigation, though I'm not sure exactly how you can have a complementary colonic irrigation, ("This tube is really fitting in quite easily, Madam. You really are most accommodating.") but they recommended I gave it a miss. I've never been so happy to follow a doctor's advice in my life!

In the last week I was there, we had the opportunity to buy any equipment we would need for our return to civilisation. I did buy just one gadget, an infra-red heat pad, which I found was very healing for the back pain I was getting intermittently (IR was very big at Hippocrates – they even had an infra-red sauna). However, I ended up not talking the pad back home with me because they couldn't supply it with a UK plug. The pad cost about $300 (which was about £200 in our money) and I did ask for a UK adaptor but by the last day it still hadn't arrived. They did offer to send it on but I wasn't going to take the risk at that stage. The whole range of gadgets was superb though – they even had a Jacuzzi you could sit in. And I knew that pain management on my return would become a big issue for me, hence my interest in the IR heat pad. While I was in the States, I was on a shedload of painkillers – I was knocking back paracetamol, ibuprofen and co-codomol like they were going out of fashion, and this was bad enough as I absolutely hate taking tablets. I was even using hot water bottles to relieve the pain in my back, the hotter the better, but they were causing bad blisters to form. But somehow I was able to complete the three weeks and come back to Merthyr.

Actually, the time passed fairly swiftly, despite my being homesick, what with missing Geraint and the kids, and being really sick what with the wheatgrass, and that was down to the people I was learning with, I think. My course lasted 21 days, but some people were there for just a week – this was pretty much like a brief introduction taster session – while others were there for a whole nine-week residential extravaganza which provided them with a certificate so that they could teach others about the Hippocrates "way".

While I was there, I came in to contact with people from all walks of life and from all over the world – though most were from states across the USA, Brazil and Europe, and from all religions  Protestants, Catholics and Jews. I spent a lot of time there with a girl from Manchester called Sonia – she is a holistic therapist here in the UK – who had lost her husband three months earlier and had come across because she was interested in learning about the course with a view to educating herself; she told me that she was hoping to come back and do the nine-week course so she could teach it herself. When I say that there were people from all walks of life, that isn't strictly true: in America, all bar the most basic healthcare costs money anyway, and Hippocrates is a private health institute.

As I've already said, homesickness was a real problem for me. In the three weeks that I was there, I ran up a £1,500 mobile phone bill – I should have bought shares in O2 – speaking to Geraint as well as the boys and my mam for ages every day. I knew his life here had become busy – he'd become Merthyr's answer to Nigella Lawson in double quick time, with three boys to feed (Zack was staying with his girlfriend Ellis) but Ger still wrote, and sent me a poem every day. It may sound soppy, but it really wasn't; it was just the sort of thing I needed to keep me going. After all, anyone can pick up a phone and talk to you when you ring them, but to actually take the time to put pen to paper (or fingers to keyboard, or thumbs to telephone) takes real effort (though Geraint has admitted he "borrowed a few", as he put it, from other poets). I've still got them too!

But family could only be on the phone for so long, and it was then that I realised how nice the people I was with really were. They could see that I was having a right old time of it, struggling as I was with homesickness as well as the pain, and they stepped in to help take me out of myself. Some of the people there were "regulars", and because they'd been before they knew just what lay a mile outside the barbed wire fence and guard towers (I'm joking of course, as we were free to come and go as we pleased). So, they were able to help organise little trips out and about, including places where we could eat raw vegetarian food so we wouldn't fall off the wagon as far as our diet was concerned. Me, I was just sorry I hadn't downloaded the McDonald's app for my iPhone before flying out to Miami, because eating out was just like being back in Hippocrates. The chef there had a really good reputation, but I felt that we were sort of eating the same things every day – I suppose on a diet that is the point – but I wish it could have been a little more varied, especially to pique my interest as I wasn't that hungry to begin with.

One night, when I was feeling really low, Sonia – the complementary therapist from Manchester – and I went to the nearest Red Lobster for a treat. Now the best way to describe the Red Lobster would be to say that it's a bit like Frankie & Benny's in terms of atmosphere and Nando's in terms of its specialisation – but while Nando's is the home of the chicken, the Red Lobster is very much the home of seafood, especially lobster. Geraint and I had been to one once before when we were in Orlando a couple of years earlier, and between us we'd eaten two delicious lobsters. And that night I had really wanted to go, but when it came down to it I just couldn't eat – Sonia ate some, but not a morsel passed my lips. I think that the smell was just too strong for me. It was something that I did learn over time: since I started suffering with cervical cancer, my sense of smell had gone into overdrive. I'm like a bloodhound on the trail of a criminal, or a shark identifying a few drops of blood in the sea; which could explain why I had such a strong reaction to the wheatgrass, as the smell turned my stomach. My reaction to the smell of food was certainly a barrier to eating it, and I lost a lot of weight in the three weeks that I was at Hippocrates.

I mentioned earlier that I had weighed 26st when I flew out; my belly was so big I needed a seatbelt extension. But by the time I came back, there was no need for the extension – the weight was literally dropping off me. I didn't weigh myself, but based on the clothes I was wearing and the way they fitted I reckon I had lost about 3st while I was in America – a stone a week, or two pounds a day – and that made 5st in total in a couple of months. I was a different woman, certainly – and Geraint proved that because, when he came to pick me up from the airport, he walked straight past me!

# Chapter Five

## From Here to Maternity

In three words I can sum up everything I've learned
about life: it goes on

*Robert Frost*

When I got back to town, after my loving husband had
totally ignored me at the airport, I discovered the
rumour machine had gone into panic mode, with
almost everyone having their own theory to explain my
absence. And for a while, the dramatic weight loss
helped me to develop an interesting cover story that I
didn't even have to lie a little bit to keep going.
Imagine the following conversation if you can:

**Local gossip 1:** "Hello Annmarie, I haven't seen
you for a long time."

**Me:** "I've been away for a couple of weeks."

**Local gossip 2:** "Have you been anywhere nice?"

**Local gossip 1:** "Yes. You've got a really nice
colour."

**Me:** "Thank you. Yes, it was a short break in
Florida."

**Local gossip 1:** "You look well. Looks like you've
lost some weight too."

**Me:** "Mmmm, Yes just a bit."

**Local gossip 2:** "Was it a good holiday? Nice posh
hotel?"

**Me:** "It wasn't a hotel; it was a health retreat

really."

And within a day, the story was everywhere: I'd gone to America to get a gastric band op! It didn't bother me at all – I know people like to talk and when they are not in full possession of the facts they will fill in the gaps with wild speculation or fibs. But I thought that this was going a bit far, even for the wildest gossips: if I wanted a gastric band done privately, wouldn't it have been easier to pop down on the train to Cardiff? Good old Merthyr – some things never change.

But some things do change. When I left Harrison, Harvey and Roddy in Geraint's tender hands, it was safe in the knowledge that they would certainly miss me while I was away. I had visions of the four of them living on takeaways, and Geraint making trips to buy more clothes rather than do the laundry. OK, I'm joking – Geraint has always been great around the house but, like all women, I like to have things done a certain way, and often it's easier to do it yourself than spending hours showing someone (and by "someone" I mean "the love of my life") how to do it. I think men know this; in fact I think men count on it. But when I got back, I was in for a real surprise – and a welcome one too. Despite never having done it before, Geraint had turned himself into something of a domestic goddess. Cooking for the boys was one thing, and I sort of expected that – I mean, he had to eat – but in addition he was now a dab hand at both the laundry AND ironing. In addition, Mam was helping out and would come up every Saturday to give all four of them a home-cooked chicken dinner with all the trimmings and gravy – and they ate it up, slice after slice. Excellent is not the word.

And things were soon back to normal, and with a vengeance. My sister Kath has only had a fleeting mention in my story so far, not least because during the vital time when things had been developing and my cancer has been diagnosed, I had kept her a bit at arms' length. I felt that she had enough to deal with on a daily basis, being pregnant with twins after having IVF treatment. If those two things were not enough, Kath was having a really difficult pregnancy and so I didn't want to add to her problems. But she now enters the story quite dramatically, and how! A couple of days after my return from Florida, I arranged to meet Kath, by now 29 weeks' pregnant, for lunch in Cowbridge, a picturesque market town in the Vale of Glamorgan where she lives. Kath took me to the Quarter Penny Café, a bistro still known universally by its former name, Farthings. I was sitting there wondering, firstly, whether what I was going to eat would meet the principles of the Hippocrates diet, and, secondly, whether I would be able to keep it down, when suddenly Kath doubled up in serious pain. A couple of minutes later she was stretched out on a banquette, moaning in agony, with me holding a pillow under her head and pretty sure that she was going into labour. I wanted to take her to the hospital where she had been getting her ante-natal care, the University Hospital of Wales in Cardiff (universally known as The Heath). But she refused, so I insisted on taking her back home, partly to get her to lie down while I phoned the hospital, but also to get a bag together just in case. She was obviously in some distress, and with twins you can't be too careful.

So I drove her back to her place and there we were, Kath lying on a bed at the top of the house and me with cervical cancer and in a lot of pain, having arrived back in the country only a couple of days earlier, running up and down the three flights of stairs and getting a bag packed. Meanwhile Kath decided she was going nowhere and started to get undressed. I got up as close to her as I possibly could, doing what the psychologists call "invading personal space", and spoke slowly and clearly: "You. Are. Going!" And that was that. We got into the car, slowly, and I started to drive down the A48 to Cardiff – I already had some experience of being a private ambulance for Dad so this was nothing new – when Kath remembered she was married. "Quick, ring Steve," she said. I used the handsfree, got hold of him and told him to meet us at Maternity in The Heath. By now Kath had become hysterical, which had been her default position for most of the day to be honest, and I was just hanging on by my fingertips trying to keep it together. For no reason a thought flashed through my mind: "What the fuck-fuck-fuck-fucking hell have I done to deserve this pile of shit?" And then just as I was starting to lose control, I saw a police patrol vehicle and started flashing my headlights to flag the driver down, with another vision, this time of driving down the middle of the road at 70mph following a police car with its "blues and two's" going like the clappers, flashing before my eyes. As the officer wound down the window, I explained the situation calmly: "Help! My sister's in labour with twins, nine weeks early and I'm ill too. Please can you get us to hospital fast?"

"You must be the unluckiest woman in Wales," said the boy in blue. "You've found the only police car in South Wales whose siren isn't working. But I'll do what I can. Follow me."

So I did get to do my high-speed flashing lights drive down into Cardiff along Cowbridge Road West – but it was more like a scene from a silent movie than *Smokey and the Bandit* – the lights were there, but the sound? Nothing. But then we drove past Ely Fire Station the policeman spied a Paramedic car and flagged it down – and, next thing you know, we got us a convoy, with the police car in the lead with its blue flashing lights, then the ambulance with its siren blaring, and finally the Range Rover carrying me and the pregnant Kath bringing up the rear. And as we drove along, Kath looked up at me, her face contorted in pain and said: "For God's sake, can you get them to turn off the siren? It's embarrassing!"

We parked up at Maternity at The Heath and I left the car and took her in – she wanted to walk but they made her go in sitting in a chair as they didn't want to take any chances. Kath was actually going into labour but doctors gave her drugs to stop the labour progressing as she was at a difficult stage of the pregnancy and had already had two false alarms.

Well, I must have been an excellent care-giver, because when I went to see her later she asked me if I'd like a job as her nanny, looking after the twins when they were finally born. I was more than a bit gobsmacked, but managed to politely decline, which was something of a surprise for me.

"There's one born every minute," Geraint said. But not me. And, on that day, not the twins either!

Three weeks later, Kath was out of hospital and doing her thing as if nothing had happened. She had gone up on the Monday to stay with Mam in Church Village, and the last thing she expected was another scare. But then on the Friday night at about 11pm Geraint and I were tucked up in bed, looking like a *Morecambe & Wise* sketch, when we got the phone call – Kath was in labour again and needed to get to Cardiff. Mam couldn't take her – it was Friday night and she was as Prosecco'd as a newt – so guess who got the call? That's right: Muggins and her private ambulance again! Steve was out with his boys at the cinema, so no matter that it was late, that I was 15 miles away, that I had four kids myself and was still a little under the weather with my own "health challenge": we were the designated drivers. My fault for being so calm last time, I suppose.

So Ger and I got up, got dressed and then went into my eldest son's room and told him: "We're off down The Heath." And 25 minutes later, we were down at Mam's in Church Village ; but it was a real palaver to load Kath and Mam into the car. One was doped up on painkillers, the other on sparkling Italian wine. Mam was so pissed she came out without putting on any make-up – she's never left the house without it in all the time I can remember. She was also clutching a kitchen roll – I never did find out why. As we drove into Cardiff, Kath suddenly remembered Steve.

"Shall I ring my husband?" she said.

"Of course you must," said I. So we rang him and arranged, once again, for him to meet us at the hospital. I was doing my best to keep everyone calm as Geraint got us into the hospital and we pulled up outside Maternity – again. Bugger the consultants; I felt like I should have had a parking space with my name on it there! Her waters had broken by now and so, en route, I had rung the hospital to tell them we were coming. However, the receptionist at Maternity said she didn't know if they had a bed available for her and, because Kath was carrying twins and, with the difficulties that this might pose, given how early they were, it was possible that we'd have to go to the nearest hospital with a specialist baby unit with an available bed. And for twins, on this Saturday morning that place was Exeter. Exeter? That would be a hard sell – Kath would hate it.

As we walked into the hospital, I took a look around and it felt just like I'd never been to Florida. I'd had the cancer diagnosis and been away, and now I was having to deal with all of this and try to be the voice of reason. Hippocrates was just a memory. When I got on that plane, I just left all my baggage behind, all the stresses and family dramas that went with it – nothing serious, just the day-to-day strains that everyone puts up with. But when I came home it was the same as before, but with extra helpings of shit to deal with.

Meanwhile, back in the real world, Kath was screaming in agony when they took her in, despite an epidural and the ubiquitous gas and air. So there we were, Kath, Mam, Geraint, Steve and I waiting in a single side room at The Heath. And at about 5am on Saturday morning, seven hours after she was first admitted, the doctors decided that they couldn't let her go on indefinitely in labour, and the decision was taken then for her to have the twins delivered by Caesarean Section. And so they were – Isabel and Daisy. But once the babies were born, neither Geraint nor I could see them. Procedures in specialist baby care units are very strict and the only people allowed in are the parents and grandparents. It's a lot like trying to get into nightclubs like Boujis in London – if your name's not on that list then you're not getting in. Other members of the family, no matter how close they are, are not covered by the protocols. But this was when Steve, showing the sharpness – and shamelessness – that makes him such a good businessman, stepped in. He went outside with the nurse and, I don't know for sure what he said to her, but all of a sudden the bouncers moved the red velvet ropes and I was allowed into the VIP section. I suspect he got out the violins and told her I was dying from cancer or something like that – I don't think he was really trying to kill me off ahead of time though!

Once the drama had settled down, we got back to normality, or whatever our normality had now become.

I was getting on with the Hippocrates diet as best I could, but there was still a cloud on the horizon. When I was out in Florida, I had found the diet difficult to come to terms with, but I thought this might have been only a temporary thing, brought on by a number of factors: the stress of being away, my abnormally well-developed sense of smell, the fact that it was something of a new departure for me as I had always been a carnivorous omnivore (I'll eat basically anything, especially when it comes with meat, poultry or fish). But that hadn't turned out to be the case at all.

Harrison was cooking some Southern Fried potato wedges, and whereas in the past that would not have bothered me at all, the smell now was so spicy and acrid that it hit the back of my throat and made me gag. And they were only potato wedges – a curry would have blown my head off at 25 yards! Even now, months on, I still have a sensitive 'nose' and garlic, in particular, turns my stomach, so whenever Geraint has something spicy – garlic prawns, Chicken Kiev or something like that – we have to sleep with a pillow between us so the smell doesn't waft into my face when he breathes on me (I still haven't worked out a barrier to block out the stink when he farts in bed, but I will!).

I couldn't go on not being able to handle the smell of food: it just wasn't practical as I didn't live alone and couldn't spend my time in isolation. I had to do something, so after the drama of Kath and the twins had settled a bit, and when I had declined her offer to sign myself up for indentured servitude (I like *Downton Abbey*, but I wouldn't want to work there), I decided to take a trip up to Manchester to see my friend from Hippocrates, Sonia. I thought it would be a good idea to take advantage of the fact that she was a therapist herself and she already knew my history from our long chats and our breakout to the Red Lobster together, and see if she could do anything to help me. And I needed help because, if anything, things had got worse. My sense of smell was now so acute and my stomach so sensitive I couldn't tolerate any of the Hippocrates foods – the tree bark, grasses and things like that. And obviously, for their therapy to work and for me to make my body "alkaline", I had to follow their eating plans – and right now, I just was not able to do that.

When Sonia saw me, she really could not believe the extent to which I was being sick, or the amount. She offered me a dry cracker that she had in her consulting rooms. "Try these, they're dry vegan," she said. But no sooner had I put it in my mouth than I had to run to the toilet because I felt sick. After I'd finished throwing up and came back into the room, she told me something that no one had picked up on. "Your sickness is psychological, completely psychological," she said. "It doesn't matter what was – or was not – in the cracker; you were sick before any of the food even entered your stomach or system. You went to America to change your diet: before you were eating everything but now you're not eating anything. It's as if you've trained your mind to just reject all food, no matter what sort."

The next step, she suggested, was to go to see a counsellor and talk through what had happened and discuss my issues with food. From there it would be a case of "reprogramming" my brain to accept food. By this time, my weight had fallen to around 20st, from a top weight of 28st, and to outsiders who weren't aware of my diagnosis – and only a very small number were – I had never been better.

I wrote earlier in my tale about how, when I went to see my consultant oncologist, Rob Howells at

Llandough hospital back in April, we had agreed that even though I was going out to Hippocrates, we would make another NHS appointment for four months down the line, after I returned from the States and had had a chance for the diet regime to bed in, to review my progress. I'm ever the optimist and really I agreed to this even though I knew it was going to be a waste of time, and the American adventure would have paid off and my cancer would have turned a corner. But having said that, I decided that I would go back to Llandough. There's no point in going into these things half-cocked, so Geraint and I also decided that, before going to see Rob, I would have another MRI scan to give him the maximum amount of information to work with.

So when we went into his consulting room that August day, Rob had everything at his fingertips. But what did he have to tell me?

## Chapter Six

### Bugger!

*Murphy's First Law:* If something can go
wrong, it will
*O'Toole's Corollary to Murphy's Law:* Murphy
was an optimist

It didn't take long for my carefully constructed sense
of optimism to be demolished, however. Sitting there
with a report in his hand and the results of my scan on
his computer monitor, Rob delivered his news as
compassionately and professionally as he possibly
could, but each piece of information was a significant
blow. Looking back, I suppose the information was
delivered very quickly, but there seemed to be such a
long pause between each fact that I had plenty of time
to speculate.

The cancer is still there. *Well of course it is, I
expected that. There was a possibility that it could
have been completely eradicated but the chances of
that were pretty slim, once I thought about it seriously,
and that would have been too much to hope for. But of
course, that doesn't mean that it has grown.*

The tumour has grown in size. *OK, well that was
always a possibility, but it's not as if it has become
more aggressive.*

The cancer is more aggressive and is now at Stage
III. *Bugger!*

When I'd last seen him, Rob had been keen for me to go down the conventional path of medical intervention and proceed with a biopsy to find out more about the pathology of my tumour, and I wouldn't have blamed him at all if he had been tempted to say "I told you so". But it was clear to me that, despite his professional "doctor's face", it was very upsetting for him to be giving me this news.

When I've talked to people about this moment since, the one thing they've all asked is: what was I thinking when I was given the news? Did I think "I should have gone with the doctor's advice and had chemotherapy or radiotherapy at once"? And the honest answer is no. I know some people may feel that I am trying to support the decision I took, but I honestly feel that Hippocrates did not fail me; if anything, I failed Hippocrates. If the dietary approach didn't work, then it didn't work because I didn't follow the programme religiously enough, and the reason for that was that I literally couldn't handle the food. Of course, another way of looking at it is to say that Hippocrates did work for me – and that if I hadn't switched to an alkali-forming diet and lifestyle, consciously moving away from the acid-forming regime that helps cancers grow, then my tumour might have grown even more than it had.

But whether I had been right or wrong in choosing not to have medical treatment immediately didn't matter any more; we were where we were, and any decisions we took had to be based on my current condition. Rob told me that he would like to have a tissue sample taken now, and recommended a biopsy: was I willing to do it? I said that I was, with the proviso that I would be wide awake when the procedure was carried out. Rob said that he didn't see any problem with that, and a week later I was back at

Llandough for the biopsy. In the next bed was an 80-year-old woman who was in for a gynaecological procedure so that she would be fit enough to undergo a hip replacement operation.

My biopsy was a same-day procedure with the results scheduled to come back in two weeks. And turn the tests round in a fortnight the scientists did. Based on what they saw I was sent to Velindre Hospital in the Cardiff suburb of Whitchurch for an ultrasound scan. In Wales, Velindre is *the* cancer hospital, where many of the senior staff are based. The scan results did not make very good reading, as it detected that the cancer had now spread to my lymph nodes.

There's a line from the film *A Good Year*, where Albert Finney's character says that you can tell you're ill when your doctor stops talking about your health and wants to talk about the weather instead. It's like your health has become the elephant in the room. And that's how it was with the ultrasound results, I think, because they did not actually tell me officially. However, I'm sure they had decided it was now at Stage IV because it had spread to another part of the body. So it did look like I'd be having some conventional medical treatments after all …

We decided that I wouldn't be making any big announcements straight away. My view was that I'd be quite happy to keep things on a need-to-know basis for as long as possible, as we had when I was originally diagnosed. Geraint's position was a little different though. He knew that because of the treatment I'd be undergoing, rugby was a no-no, and he'd have to effectively give up coaching his beloved team which, over a period of years, he had developed into one of the strongest in Wales, because he couldn't drop out half way through. Not only that, but his decision was made more difficult by the fact that Harvey was in the team. Now the way age-grade rugby in Wales tends to be organised at most clubs is that a group of coaches take on a team at the beginning of their playing careers, when the boys are aged eight or nine, and take them through their development up until Youth rugby. And while this can lead to problems from a playing point of view, with coaches and players getting too used to one another, from a social aspect it is great because you become like a group of friends, a Tuesday night and Sunday morning family almost. And for this reason he knew he'd have to tell a few of the coaches why he was dropping out – better for Geraint to explain it to them and ask them to keep the confidence than have them asking if something was wrong and speculating. That way we could manage the news ourselves.

But, to some extent, even though we did not want my cancer to become a sort of sideshow, the question of what to say, and to whom, was a little bit like rearranging the deckchairs on the Titanic. The big question to answer now was what sort of treatment regimen should I follow? The course of treatment Rob Howells outlined was a two-pronged attack on my tumour and the lymph nodes which had become cancerous. Prong 1 was a five-week course of external radiotherapy, with five treatments each week; this would then be followed by a less frequent course of internal radiotherapy. Prong 2 was chemotherapy, in Rob's view ideally involving two drugs: carboplatin and paclitaxel. Now each type of chemotherapy comes with its own book, telling you all about the treatment, the potential upsides and downsides, as well as the technical details – the "how, what, when and where" if you like. Now I don't think everyone likes to get stuck into that amount of detail – it can make your cancer that much more real, whereas if you just listen to a doctor telling you about the available treatments you can almost pretend that it's not happening to you. But as you can probably guess, I like to do research so I took all the books and read them carefully before making any decisions. Because I had all the information in front of me, I think that it will be easier for you to understand how I made the decisions I did, if I tell you a little about each of the treatments.

Radiotherapy involves using high energy X-rays and similar rays to treat the disease. Radiotherapy works by destroying cancer cells in the area that is being treated by radiation. However, normal cells can also be damaged by radiotherapy, though they usually repair themselves. With some types of cancer, radiotherapy can cure the cancer and can also reduce the chance of its recurring after surgery. It may also be used to control a cancer or to help improve the symptoms of it.

Radiotherapy is used as part of many patients' cancer treatment, and can be given either as external radiotherapy (from outside the body using high energy X-rays) or as internal radiotherapy (when a radioactive material is actually placed within the body). It was proposed that I would have both.

External radiotherapy is normally given as a series of short, daily treatments in the radiotherapy department using equipment similar to a large X-ray machine, and this was what Rob Howells was proposing as the first part of my radiotherapy treatment. Treatment is individually planned, so people with the same type of cancer may have different types of treatment. A course of treatment may last from as little as a fortnight to seven weeks – in my case, five weeks was proposed. The treatments are usually given once a day (though in some cases two treatments a day are scheduled), with the weekends left free for the body to recover. Each treatment is called a fraction. Giving the treatment in fractions ensures that less damage is done to normal cells than to cancer cells. The damage to normal cells is mainly temporary, but this is what causes the side-effects of radiotherapy. Usually, each radiotherapy treatment takes about 10–15 minutes. Most of this time is spent getting you in position and doing checks, and the treatment itself normally only lasts a few minutes. Radiotherapy treatment for most cancers, apart from skin cancers, is delivered by a linear accelerator. The treatment itself is painless, although it may gradually cause some side-effects.

Internal radiotherapy is used mainly to treat cancers in the cervix and womb, as well as in the head and neck area, the prostate or skin. It can either be given by brachytherapy, where the medics put solid radioactive material close to or inside the tumour for a short period of time, or by what is called radioisotope treatment, where a radioactive liquid is given as a drink or is injected into a vein. Brachytherapy was the type of internal radiotherapy that I would have, should I choose to go down that route, and it would mean that I would only need to stay in isolation while the radioactive source was in place. Once it has been removed, the radioactivity disappears and it would be perfectly safe to be with other people (however, people with prostate cancer who receive brachytherapy do not have the radioactive seeds removed, but because the radiation affects an area of only a few millimetres around the seeds, there's no danger of other people being affected by the radiation).

As for the chemotherapy drugs, carboplatin is usually given to treat ovarian and lung cancer, but may also be used to treat many other types of cancer such as mine, and it is normally given alongside other chemotherapy drugs as a combination treatment. Carboplatin is a colourless fluid which can be given as a drip in a number of ways – as a cannula (through a fine tube inserted into a vein, usually in the back of the hand), as a central line (through a fine, plastic tube inserted under the skin and into a vein near the collarbone) or as a PICC line (into a fine tube inserted into a vein in the crook of the arm). The infusion takes about an hour to complete, and the drug is usually given as a course of several sessions (cycles) of treatment over a few months, with the length of treatment and the number of cycles depending on the type of cancer.

The big downside of any chemotherapy is the side-effects; there are a number of main ones and there is no way of telling which one or ones you might have, and if you're having a combination treatment, there could be other side-effects. One big side effect is the risk of infection: carboplatin can reduce the number of white blood cells which are produced in the bone marrow, and if the number of white blood cells is low (a condition doctors call neutropenia), you are more likely to pick up infections. The risk of contracting infections is greatest around 10–14 days after chemotherapy, before the number of white cells starts to increase again and become normal before the next cycle of chemo; blood tests will confirm this is the case, and if it doesn't the next cycle may be delayed. Carboplatin can also reduce the production of platelets, which help the blood to clot, so there may be unexplained bruising or bleeding, like nosebleeds, bleeding gums, blood spots or rashes on the skin (in some cases, it may be necessary to give a platelet transfusion). Another possible side effect is anaemia, as carboplatin can reduce the number of red blood cells which carry oxygen around the body; this may make you feel tired and breathless. Sickness and loss of appetite are possible side-effects and usually last no more than a day (sickness) or a couple of days (loss of appetite). Anti-sickness drugs may help stop or reduce nausea. The most frequently seen side-effect is tiredness, especially towards the end of treatment and for some weeks afterwards. The only way to deal with this is to rest and take some gentle exercise. The tiredness can impact on your ability to work though, making it unsafe to drive or operate machinery – but because I was not working, this had less impact on me than it would have on others.

In addition to these main side-effects, some others are seen less often: these include numbness or tingling in the hands or feet (caused by carboplatin's effect on nerves), changes in hearing (possibly tinnitus or not being able to hear some high-pitched sounds), diarrhoea and constipation, sore or dry mouth or food tasting funny. In some extreme cases, the kidneys may be affected though this doesn't usually cause any symptoms and the effect is generally mild, but if the effect is severe, the kidneys can be permanently damaged unless the treatment is stopped (if you undergo chemotherapy, blood tests will check kidney function before each treatment). Hair loss is extremely rare with normal doses of carboplatin but can happen with high-dose treatment; this may begin three or four weeks after starting treatment although it can start sooner, but it is temporary and hair will start to grow back once treatment ends.

Paclitaxel (also known as Taxol) is usually given to treat ovarian, breast and non-small cell lung cancer, and is made from extracts of the yew tree. Like carboplatin, it is a colourless fluid and is administered in the same way. Many of the main side effects of paclitaxel are also those found in carboplatin: an increased risk of infection, bruising or bleeding, anaemia, sickness and tiredness. In addition however it has a number of other side-effects. Some of these are also the less often seen side-effects of carboplatin, like numbness and tingling in the hands and feet, sore mouth and taste changes, diarrhoea and hair loss (though with paclitaxel, this can happen after only two or three weeks), but some are just paclitaxel-related.

Some people can have an allergic reaction to paclitaxel while it is being given; symptoms of this may include skin rashes and itching, a high temperature, shivering, dizziness, headaches and breathlessness. Paclitaxel may also cause aches in joints and muscles (though these will normally pass within a few days), a rash or dry skin patches (which may be itchy) and headaches. Sometimes paclitaxel can cause pain along the vein that is used to deliver the chemotherapy. Less common side-effects of paclitaxel include low blood pressure, temporary slowing in the heart rate (bradycardia), temporary (usually) changes in the way the liver works and abdominal pain.

A further potential risk to health is the possibility of developing blood clots, which may be increased by having chemotherapy. Paclitaxel is incredibly toxic, so side by side with the health risks of having it is the benefit that it should actually kill everything that needs to be killed. However, in real life it doesn't always work out like that – I know of one woman who has cervical cancer and used paclitaxel and had the same end-result as me. Not everyone is the same. It became clear to me, as I read the books and thought about the people I know who have had cancer and the treatments they underwent, that with cancer there are no guarantees. So it all came down to gut instinct, I'm afraid.

Overall, when I looked at the treatment options, the

radiotherapy seemed like a no-brainer; I had to do that. The more I looked at the chemotherapy, though, the more risky and severe it sounded. So I asked my oncology consultant at Velindre, Louise Hanna, what change could I expect to make to my life expectancy if I went down the chemotherapy route, as well as having radiotherapy. She said that the chemotherapy could give me a 10% chance of extending my life. Now that's not increasing my life expectancy by 10% – but just one chance in ten of increasing it at all. So that answer, combined with the risks, side effects and what I saw as a general reduction in the quality of my life persuaded me. I decided to go for just radiotherapy – the chemo would have to wait, and I'd see if I needed it.

There was one potential side-effect from chemotherapy that did seem like a real benefit to me, however, and that was that my incredibly strong sense of smell might well be kicked back into sync, so I'd be able to eat food again, and get back on with the Hippocrates diet. But that would need to be shelved for now.

## Chapter Seven

### Here We Go

Today we fight. Tomorrow we fight. The day after, we
fight. And if this disease plans on whipping us, it better
bring a lunch, 'cause it's gonna have
a long day doing it.

*Jim Beaver*

The next two months saw me visiting hospital more
times on my own behalf than I had done in the rest of
my lifetime. The external radiotherapy course of
treatment I was scheduled to undergo at Velindre
Hospital was effectively a five-week intensive blast of
radiation. The following three weeks saw me having
radioactive material inserted into my vagina once a
week.

Now it's time for another one of those annoying
medical bits, where I get to explain what happened to
me in more detail. In the last chapter, I talked about
radiation generally but now it's time to get into what
really happens, so you can get a feel for what was
going through my mind when I underwent the
treatment.

The five-week course of external radiation was
fairly straightforward. Basically, I got up onto a table
in the same room as the linear accelerator, and the
radiographers positioned me on the table and adjusted
its height and position. Because it's so important to get

the patient into the correct position, the radiographers can take a little while to get this just right. The table itself is quite hard, but there are foam pads and pillows available to make patients as comfortable as possible so they are less likely to move and fidget. And it was important for me to be as still as possible while the radiotherapy was being delivered. Once I was correctly lined up, the radiographers would get out of the room, leaving me alone while the treatment took place, so that they were not exposed to any unnecessary radiation.

One thing does seem a bit strange, though, but, when you think about it, makes a lot of sense. The final step before the radiographers began to give me external radiotherapy was to tattoo a mark so that they could ensure they were treating the exact same spot every time, then future treatments could be set up faster and with less fuss. So, at the relatively advanced age of 43, I would be having my first tattoo. At last, I thought, I can say: "I really am a Merthyr girl!"

As far as the internal radiotherapy is concerned, the aim of the brachytherapy is to deliver radiation directly to the cervix and the area close by, with the radioactive material put in place using a brachytherapy machine which delivers the source material through specially designed hollow tubes called applicators. There are two types of brachytherapy that you can have, depending on whether you've had a hysterectomy or not. Patients who have not had hysterectomies undergo intra-uterine brachytherapy. In this procedure, a doctor inserts the applicators into the vagina and passes them up through the cervix into the womb. Sometimes additional applicators are placed alongside the cervix.

In normal circumstances, the applicators are inserted in an operating room while you're sedated or under a general anaesthetic, though an epidural may also be used. To prevent the applicators moving, a pack of cotton/gauze padding is placed inside the vagina, and sometimes a piece of gauze is also placed inside your bum, and you may have a catheter put into your bladder to drain off urine. Painkillers are normally given to ease any discomfort. (For patients who have had a hysterectomy, intravaginal brachytherapy is performed. In this case, a single larger hollow tube applicator is placed in the vagina. With intravaginal brachytherapy you don't need an anaesthetic or sedation to insert the applicator and padding isn't necessary.)

Once the applicators have been placed in the exact spot – the alignment of which is aided by tattoos which have already been inked in – an MRI scan, a CT scan or X-ray is carried out to confirm that they have been placed exactly right. Once that has been confirmed, they are connected to the brachytherapy machine which then delivers the radioactive source into the applicators and administers the radiotherapy treatment.

Brachytherapy may be given in several short bursts or in one long slow treatment, depending on the systems used.

High dose rate treatment is the most common way of giving brachytherapy to the cervix in the UK. With high dose rate treatment, a high dose of radioactivity produced from iridium or cobalt is delivered over a few minutes. Usually the treatment takes about 10–15 minutes and is repeated several times, a few days apart. For example, you may have treatment four times over several days while you're an in-patient. The applicators are usually removed between treatments, but in a few hospitals they're left in place between treatments and then removed after the final treatment. Alternatively the treatment may be given as an outpatient or day case on three or four occasions over several days or weeks. This was the treatment I had, and it was a once-a-week treatment for three weeks.

Low dose rate treatment is usually given over a period of 12–24 hours as an inpatient, but sometimes it may be given over a few days. The applicators are usually left in place until the treatment has finished. Patients receiving low dose treatment are normally kept in bed to make sure that the applicators stay in the right place, and also have a catheter fitted. Because leaving the applicators in place can be uncomfortable, regular strong doses of painkillers tend to be given until the treatment has finished and the applicators are removed.

Another type of treatment is pulsed dose rate brachytherapy, in which the applicators stay in place for the same length of time as low dose rate treatment, but the radiation dose is given in pulses rather than as a continuous low dose.

In my case, because I've not had a hysterectomy, I was going to be given high dose rate intra-uterine brachytherapy. Now Velindre had never had a patient who wanted to be awake during the procedure before and when I went to meet up with Louise Hanna, we hit a glitch – again. When she was examining me prior to my having the epidural, she noticed my back wasn't clear. There were blemishes and what looked like pus-filled pockets under the skin (this was a side effect of the external radiotherapy). Both she and her anaesthetist looked at it to decide whether it was safe for them to administer the epidural, and whether they could pass a needle in between all the sores. In the end, they decided that it was far too risky to attempt an epidural as the potential downsides more than outweighed the benefits of trying. In the worst case, an infected needle passing into the spinal cord could well cause paralysis. "Ah well," says I. "Can't be helped.

I'll wait a week for the infection to clear up and then I'll come back and have it." But both Louise Hanna and the gas-passer wanted to push on. My medical condition generally was one reason for them wanting to go on and begin the radiotherapy as soon as possible, but another consideration – and quite a valid one too, I had to admit – was that neither of them had come across a skin infection like mine before: they didn't know what it was and, frankly, didn't know if it would be clear in a week so even if we waited, we might well be in the same position.

So the only option for them was my big no-no – the general anaesthetic. Not surprisingly, I was dead against it – I'd never had a general anaesthetic before and both my sister and dad had suffered reactions when they had been put under. Add to that the fact that I have high blood pressure and you can probably understand why I didn't want to go through it, and this was what I explained this to the anaesthetist. The only other option as far as he could see was a local anaesthetic, but he said that before approving it we'd need to speak to Louise as she would be the one performing the procedure. This would be new ground for her – she'd never done this just using a local before, but I thought I was making a good case: I'd had four children, all without pain relief, so I knew my pain threshold was high, and I told her that I'd be more than willing to give it a go if she would, and the anaesthetist would also be there in support if needed. However, I could see it was going to be a big ask – after all, the procedure would take up to two and a half hours and that was a long time for me to be immobile with my feet up in stirrups while not under anaesthetic.

I don't think Louise was best pleased at my suggestion, but she said that she was prepared to give it a shot too, so in we went. And looking back, I can see why they want to use a general anaesthetic, or at the very least an epidural, because it really was traumatic and certainly more painful than having the four kids. The hard part was placing the applicators, and this required my stomach to be probed forcefully by an ultrasound machine, operated by a tiny radiologist named Polly. And God, was she forceful! "Polly, you may be small but you're deadly," I told her. She was shocked to be told she was rough –because 95% of the patients she did this to were completely unconscious, and the other 5% were comfortably numb because they'd had an epidural, she'd probably never had a complaint before. But I always like to be first.

Then they put the applicators in place – from the ultrasound they looked to be in the right spots but they had to do a CT scan to be sure, so they then they had to wheel me through the corridor in probably the most unflattering position you can imagine – and if you can't, then think of a turkey on Christmas Eve just before you get on with loading the stuffing. I expressed some concern about my modesty. "Don't worry," they said. "We'll have security on the doors." Visions of the bouncers from outside the Kirkhouse, a well-known Merthyr drinking establishment and nightspot, flashed through my mind but thankfully that was not what they meant.

I suppose I should have been honoured really – normally the only time they do this sort of thing is when someone has died and they have to move the body to the mortuary. They covered me in a sheet – not over my face, no – and then about ten people walked me through to the CT room. It's a bit like being the President of the United States with the Secret Service running next to the car. Except that instead of dark suits and ties, they wear surgical scrubs. Someone – a female nurse I think – held the door open for the bed, and I smiled up at her and said "Thanks". The girl jumped out of her skin, and I said: "You have a live one tonight." Recovering, the nurse said: "I wasn't expecting to see you with your eyes open!"

The CT showed that the applicators were in the right spot, so they wheeled me back to the treatment room and hooked my applicators up to the brachytherapy machine, and started to run it to administer the radiotherapy. After about 15–20 minutes, they had administered the first dose of radiation and I was unhooked and whipped back into theatre so they could remove the applicators. Then I was wheeled into recovery, but I really didn't need to recover. I hadn't had any real sort of anaesthetic to snap out of. I had a coffee and another CT scan to ensure everything was fine, and then I was taken back to the ward. They wanted me to hang around another two or three hours but by this time I was up, dressed and ready to go, tapping my feet against the chair legs. And as soon as I could, I was gone. The local anaesthetic certainly helped a bit in taking the edge off the pain, but even so there were a few "grit your teeth" moments while the applicators were being placed. But overall it went pretty well, I'd say.

Looking back, my rush to get out certainly helped establish my reputation for being a bit … well in a hurry, shall we say? I don't like to hang about. When most people give blood, they wait until they go to the hospital for the test results – when I do it, I ask them to ring me as soon as they have them back so we can crack on. The first time I asked them to do that, Louise Hanna said: "We don't normally do that sort of thing, but I will for you, because it's obvious you're a VIP."

"Yes," I said, "a VIP – a very impatient person." And that's me.

The course of treatment finished on November 25 –

a date that's easy to remember as it is Mam and Dad's wedding anniversary – and I had a consultation booked for January 5. It was all very breezy and almost jokey. When I walked onto her consulting room, Louise Hanna said: "You're looking really relaxed."

"Yes," I said. "I feel absolutely great. Being pain-free is such a huge thing after being in constant discomfort for almost a year." We booked a scan for the beginning of March, with an appointment to discuss the results on March 15 – a date which we took to be a good omen as it was Dad's birthday. (Everything seemed to be happening on the anniversary of something or other, and in between, on March 8 – Roddy's birthday – we moved house, transplanting all the family from our home in Merthyr to a barn conversion in a little village on the outskirts of Brecon.)

The March 15 results consultation went well. Everything seemed to be shrinking and we were very pleased with the outcome, as was Louise Hanna. We booked another scan and consultation for June and, looking forward to even more good news, started to get on top of our new home.

# Chapter Eight

## The Barn

Turn it into something good
### *Annmarie James-Thomas*

I've always set myself targets. Perhaps it's partly because of feeling a little bit psychic, but I have always found myself confronted by goals to achieve – and I always achieve them. I have had a vision board for many years, on which I pin notes about the things I want to achieve. They always happen, though not always in the way you might expect them to.

One such aspiration was my wanting to live in a barn – not in a cows and horses sort of way, but in a nicely designed, well-laid out converted barn. I wasn't sure how or when it would happen, but on the vision board it went.

Then lo and behold, about two years ago, I was reading one of the *Sunday Times* supplements and saw an advertisement: the BBC – or more accurately a production company looking to make a series on its behalf – was looking for couples to design and build their dream home for a game show. The idea of the series was for couples to take a derelict or disused building and convert it into their dream dwelling, taking into account external and interior design, location and so on. Six couples would then be chosen to take part in the actual series, with programmes following through their vision from beginning to end. The production company would acquire the properties and engage builders, plumbers, electricians and a whole range of tradesmen to bring the projects to fruition. The couple who designed and project managed the winning project, chosen either by the public or a panel of judges, would win their dream home.

I didn't think any more about it, but then one wet Sunday afternoon – everyone knows the joke that the worst place to be is Merthyr on a wet Sunday afternoon, because the pubs are shut – we decided to go for a drive, so Geraint and I drove along the A470 out of Merthyr and headed up to Brecon. The A470 runs along a valley between the two towns; at the highest point in the valley floor is the Storey Arms adult education centre, and as we drove past the weather began to change rapidly. Back towards Merthyr the rain continued to fall, but up towards Brecon we could see blue skies and sunshine. We got to Brecon and as we drove past the Golf Club, we saw a sign that read "Barns for sale". We bought the ice-creams we'd driven up for, then went back and took a look. The farmyard we came to had two barns, both derelict, and I loved them. I could see how they might look in the future, renovated and developed, and thought they would make a great home – not only that but the location and views were incredible with Pen-y-Fan, the highest peak in the Brecon Beacons, dominating the skyline.

When we came home, we got on to the computer and found the website of the estate agent handling the sale and saw it could easily be the dream home that I had always wanted. The price was a little steep, though – it was listed at £300,000 for the barn in the state it was in; I reckoned it would cost as much again to renovate. There was no way we could afford to do it – so it looked like the dream home would have to stay on the vision board until my lottery numbers came up. But then I remembered the *Sunday Times* advert for the BBC television series, and the dream looked doable once more.

The estate agents already had planning permission for the barn, and a plan to renovate it. I got hold of a copy but decided I didn't like it and wanted to do my own instead. So, I emailed the production company and pitched my idea for a barn conversion in rural Powys. They replied and said that if I could give them more details, along with some photographs of the barn as it was and sketches of how we wanted it to look then they would take a look and consider our proposal further. I got out my sketch book and started roughing out some Annmarie impressions of the finished project, scanned them in and sent them back to the producers. They got back in touch, asking for a contact number and then a couple of the researchers rang us and talked through the idea in more detail. A couple more to-and-fro conversations and they pretty much knew what we were thinking about, and by now we had refined our plans too. By this time, however, Dad had died and one of my abiding regrets was that he would have loved what we were trying to do with the place, and had he been well enough he certainly would have helped us with it.

Soon, the producers were in touch – we seemed to have got onto a shortlist because they wanted to come with a film crew to see the location and film some footage of Geraint and I at the place, along with some or all of the boys, so that they could have an introductory piece about our project if we made the final cut and got to be one of the six couples. Thankfully, the barn was still on the market so we approached the agents and asked for permission to bring the crew to the barn and film. The place had been on the market for a while, so we thought that any interest would have been welcome, but the agent said no – apparently the owner wouldn't have it. Once more, our bubble seemed to have been punctured by an unwelcome prick, but we rang the production company – they'd been decent with us so it was only fair to let them know so that they didn't waste their time on us. But then we had a good surprise. "No problem," said the producers. "Find another barn to film at – any derelict barn will do."

I remembered that my sister Kath and her husband Steve have a barn up near Usk, and they said we could film there. So having got the location, we invited the film crew and producers over. I'm going all out to impress now, so I thought laying on a picnic was the right thing to do – not for us a pie and a pint in one of the local pubs. The spot for the picnic was recce'd too – in the end we decided on the top of Usk Mountain – and then I gave some thought to the menu. In addition to the traditional picnic fare, in case the "meejah types" were vegetarians, I even catered a veggie option – in this case brie and grape baguettes. The interview on camera went well: they asked Geraint questions and I answered – and they thought it was hilarious. Then they filmed Geraint and the boys having a kick-about with a football in the field in front of the barn. We thought we were in with a good chance after they said, as they were leaving, that we'd hear by December. If we got that far, the next task, they said, would be to build a scale model of our project so there would be something visual to work with in the early stages of the programme, and allow the reality to compare with the vision. Their last words about the model were "Don't do anything yet," but their words fell on deaf ears.

Making a model! Now I was in my element – not for nothing was I *Blue Peter*'s biggest fan with my own secret supply of sticky-back plastic. I started on it straight away and it was a classic – an external view of the barn with an upstairs and downstairs you could see by lifting the roof off. The rooms were decorated, the bathroom plumbed and even the garden landscaped. I took photographs of all the elevations and emailed it to the producers in January 2011. They loved it. But the programme was being delayed.

By now, life had other plans for me and I was starting to feel ill, so not being able to proceed was not as big a blow as it might have been. However, the show had not been cancelled, the production company hastened to assure us; it was only being temporarily shelved and as soon as it was back on the production slate they would be in touch. As it turned out, of course, had the programme gone ahead I would not have been able to go through with it and that would have been awful, both for the programme and also for the family as it would have just been another load of pressure on top of us. We went up to Brecon again, in February time, and the barn was still for sale. When we first saw it, I had said to Geraint: "That barn was waiting for us." And now all that was left of that dream was the scale model I'd made for the TV programme – it's still sitting in the store room of my mother's shop in Merthyr.

While I was out in the States, word came through from the production company: the show had been cancelled. No longer on stop: it just wasn't going to happen. I was a bit sad naturally, but my mind was definitely on other things I think. Geraint and I talked about it on one of our long £1,500-bill phone calls and agreed that the property downturn had probably knocked the programme for a couple of reasons:

people might not have been so interested in the subject at this time, and the production company, which would have had to shell out for the derelict buildings up front, might have found it hard to unload the "losing" properties after the programme was filmed and not be able to realise their initial investment and costs for a while.

Nothing much happened while I was undergoing radiotherapy; moving was the last thing on my mind. But just before Christmas, we saw an advertisement for another barn conversion for sale up near Brecon. I'd just finished the treatment and I needed a lift – remember we hadn't had the results of the post-treatment scan then – so the thought of doing something normal and nice, like looking at a barn even if we couldn't afford it, was something to look forward to, so we rang the estate agent and made an appointment to view.

On the day of the viewing, we arrived early and the estate agent wasn't there yet, so the owner let us in herself. We could see immediately that it was lovely. Whereas the first barn was derelict and very much something for the future, this barn – which was named Rhiwlas – had already been converted and finished to an incredibly high standard; and as we sat there, I began mentally slotting our furnishings into place – the sofas here, the coffee table there, Fortnum & Mason hamper in that spot. Then the estate agent arrived and introduced himself: "Mr and Mrs Thomas, I'm sorry to have kept you waiting. My name is Roy." Roy! My dad's name. You could have knocked me down with a feather.

Dates and names which have symbolism and significance tend to crop up in my life – and my mam's and my nan's – like signs, and this was an omen – a good omen: Dad was watching and was somehow part of the process. It made it feel ... well, it made it feel right. And I knew this was the barn for us. Another sign was outside the window: the neighbours had a Citroën DS3, just like our son, Zack, so we asked about them, and they sounded like a very interesting couple: one runs an adventure holiday company and the other runs a car rally company and drives the DS3. It was starting to feel like we really fitted in there. A third coincidence was that Rhiwlas's owner was a holistic therapist and had set up her own treatment room in the barn. Now, having gone through cancer and with all the holistic therapies I had been through, to actually find a place with its very own treatment room was just too spooky for words.

Logistically it was perfect – the right number of bedrooms and bathrooms for the whole family, as well as a great open kitchen and lovely sitting rooms. The garden was bigger than we were used to, and normally Geraint's first move whenever we get into a new place is to lay a surface in the back – but somehow I could tell from his face that he wasn't going to be doing that here. In fact, for a pair of townies – if you can think of people who lived virtually their whole lives at the foot of the Brecon Beacons as being townies – then we were really hooked on the place, both the property itself and the location. And it wasn't as if it's too far from civilisation – the boys could continue to commute to school (it is only a half-hour drive from Merthyr) and Mam's shop was close and Cardiff is only an hour away.

We came home and talked – and decided that we really wanted to do this, so we moved fast. The barn is pretty spacious, and most of our stuff fitted in easily enough. However some things had been bought specifically for our house in Merthyr and just would not go with the size and shape of rooms, or the architecture, so a garage sale got rid of most of the bits and bobs which we could not slot in. Everything that was left went to the local charity shops.

Once we'd moved in, we quickly settled into a daily routine that worked for us and accommodated Geraint, the children, me and any treatments I might be having. On an average day, the alarm goes off at about 6.45am. Geraint gets up and takes Lulu out for her early morning walk, before coming back and making my breakfast and bringing it up to me in bed.

Then he wakes the boys up for school and makes their breakfast before diving into our bathroom for a shower and shave. They eat and get ready to set off for Merthyr by about 7.45am. While this has been going on I've got myself up, washed and dressed and I'm ready to go with them for the school run.

We get to Merthyr about 8.20am and drop Roddy and Harrison into Cyfarthfa and then head up to Mam's shop for coffee and a light second breakfast. At about 8.50, Geraint will drop Harvey into Merthyr College then come up back to the shop. We'll have a coffee and then what happens next depends on the day. If I have a therapy session or a doctor's or hospital appointment we will do that, or maybe some shopping and having my hair done. Time passes quickly because by 3pm it's time to pick the kids up from school and college, but what happens then depends on what day it is. On Mondays, Wednesdays and Fridays, Roddy and Harvey stay in Merthyr and train with one of the local boxing trainers at the Merthyr Ex-Servicemen's Club, so Geraint will drop them off and then take Harrison and me home, make tea and then come back to Merthyr to watch the end of their training sessions and bring them back to the barn. Once he's made tea for them and a snack for Harrison, himself and me, if I haven't prepared something for them in advance, then it's after 8pm.

I will normally have gone up to bed soon after we have come back from Merthyr at tea time, because the pain in my left leg – I've got a bit ahead of myself here chronologically, and I'll tell you about my leg pain later – is best coped with if I'm lying down. So when Geraint comes up, we will watch TV lying on the bed with Geraint massaging my leg from buttock to ankle to ease the pain. I'll speak to Mam around 9.30pm on the phone, or Avalon or one of the girls and by about 10.30pm we're completely shattered and it's time to switch the lights off, knowing that tomorrow we'll be repeating the same pattern again.

Now this may sound quite boring and repetitive – the Brecon version of *Groundhog Day*, in fact – but if you just take out the bit where I have cancer and Geraint stays at home to look after me, repetitive lives are what the vast majority of us lead. So there's no need to feel sorry for us. We're doing exactly what is necessary for us for now while I am going for treatment. And doing it in some of the nicest scenery in the world, in the home we always dreamed of.

So that's the life we live in Rhiwlas – not an imaginary life in a fairytale barn, but the real one. It's funny how things happen though. The original barn has come back on the market – it looks like the sale fell through. The model remains in my mam's shop, and I think that one day I would like to renovate my own barn – don't get me wrong, where we are now is lovely but it was designed by someone else. The one we do from scratch would be ours. But that was something to think about for the future – right now we were living the dream in Brecon.

But while we were living the dream, real life chose that very moment to kick in with a vengeance, and gave us a swift boot up the bum.

# Chapter Nine

## When I Thought I Was Out, It Pulled Me Back in …

It's déjà vu all over again

*Yogi Berra*

On June 21 2012, we celebrated our 20th wedding anniversary – another significant date. The same day, we went back to Velindre for the results of the latest scan and tests. The scan had been done at the beginning of June and, up until then there had been no obvious cause for concern. But maybe there was, because in the back of my mind was a nagging feeling that this news was not going to be as good as we were hoping for; and I wasn't feeling the same sense of positivity about this particular appointment coinciding with a family anniversary. Outwardly I was still radiating positivity and calm and there was no way I'd have admitted my doubts at the time to anyone, not even to Geraint, but deep down I just knew that it wasn't going to go well.

Why I felt like that at the time I don't really know, but now, looking back, I can see exactly when the clouds, even though there were only a few of them at first, had begun to appear on the horizon. I'd taken a tumble over the Christmas break, and this was perhaps the start of things not going right. I'd gone down to

Cowbridge with the family on New Year's Eve to see my sister during the day, and had tripped in the street and almost got run over as I fell into the path of an oncoming car. I was quite shaken, and my back and left leg were very sore. We had planned to go out that evening to see in the New Year with Jeremy and Annette Callaghan, who were having a party in Merthyr, but I was not in the right frame of mind to enjoy it, I was aching so much. But, I said to myself, it's just a bad fall. It will clear up soon once the bruising has gone down.

But it didn't get any better, so after a month when the pain was still with me, I went to see a chiropractor. During the consultation, I told her that the pain was not going away; in fact, the more I thought about it, it seemed to be getting worse. It seemed to be far worse when I moved – it was like a sciatica pain that shot down my leg. I had a couple of sessions with the chiropractor, but nothing seemed to be happening, and she said herself: "By now, we should have seen a significant improvement. If this continues, perhaps we should get an MRI scan to see what is happening there." Geraint and I talked about it, but we decided not to go down that route. After all, I said to myself, I'll be having an MRI in June just before I go back for the review with Louise Hanna, so there's no need to go privately and have one now – anything that it could pick up will be on the scan then too.

So, when we went down to see Louise, there would be two things to talk about: the tumour and my back. And still the nagging doubt in the back of my mind …

"It's not good news at all, I'm afraid," was how Louise broke the news to us. "The tumour has spread and now it's pressing against the kidneys and the uterus." Now this was a shock – I'd not been having any difficulties in passing water, in fact quite the opposite, and my urine seemed fine. But the next things she told us suddenly made all the pieces of my post-New Year jigsaw fit together. Not only was the tumour pressing against the kidneys and uterus, but it was also pressing on the sciatic nerve and this was probably the cause of the pains that continued to radiate up and down my back and legs.

The options Louise outlined were pretty much the same as last time – and they were both chemotherapy. And once again, I was confronted with the same choice of chemo as before: carboplatin and paclitaxel – either, both or neither? This time, however, there was a third option on the table: to take part in a clinical trial. So I had to weigh the choices and make a decision. Well let's get the vanity out of the way first: as far as the carboplatin/paclitaxel choice went, one factor I might want to take into account was hair loss. One does not make your hair fall out (carboplatin) but the other one (paclitaxel) does. The hair loss was not an issue for me – I've always worn hats and hair scarves and the wigs you can get are fantastic. Another factor that helped me reach my decision was just as personal, but – to my mind – far more logical: as soon as I heard the word "paclitaxel" I said to myself "nope, not having that" because that was the course of chemotherapy my father had. And by the end it had laid him just as low as the cancer had, and to what end?

The clinical trial option was not as good as it sounded either. What if, with my high blood pressure, I couldn't get selected? Or if I did, might the treatment not kill me within two weeks? Another drawback was the very nature of clinical trials; it is a trial and to test whether the drug or treatment is working, a similarly sized sample of people must be given a placebo to compare the condition of people who take the drug with those who do not. So if you end up in the control group then you will get no treatment at all, and while we can all see the value of the testing process, no one wants to be in the control group. So with the drug trial, there is a 50–50 chance of not receiving any drug at all – and that's before you factor in the chances of it working. I like the odds on the National Lottery better. Okay, they're not really better, but the consequences of winning the lottery or not are life-changing, but not life-threatening.

Whichever option I chose, however, the chemotherapy was toxic and could, in the case of paclitaxel, actually be cancerous itself, so the treatment came with its own risks. Not only that, but whichever option I chose would lead to a reduction in my quality of life while I was receiving it – I'd have less energy for sure. But these were just complicating factors: I had to choose something. So, after weighing up the pros and cons I opted for carboplatin chemotherapy only, the least risky – to my mind – of the options open to me. This would be a rolling course of treatment, with one chemo being administered every three weeks. But before I could start having treatment, Louise Hanna said that I would need to undergo an operation to fit a stent, because the tumour was pressing on the left kidney. She contacted the urologist and said that we'd need to get this done as soon as possible, because chemo could not begin without the operation. They did a kidney function test first, to ensure everything was working fine – the results came back OK, but I wasn't really expecting anything else as, whatever was going on with the rest of my body, my bladder was filling and emptying like clockwork.

The journey back from Velindre was occupied with more planning. Mam was away on a Rhine cruise – well that's where she thought she was going – so we decided to tell her when she came back rather than give her the news over the phone. Apart from not wanting to spoil her holiday, it wasn't as if we could do anything about it. Now the story of Mam's cruise along the Rhine is worth sharing. She'd booked to go with some friends, and in the week leading up to her departure she went to Cardiff and bought an excellent German phrase book and had practised so that she was perfectly able to order her Riesling with only a trace of a Welsh accent. We went to see her a day or so before she was going in order to get contact details, numbers and so on, the way you do; and while we were there, Geraint started looking at the itinerary and he began to read out loud: "First it's the Eurostar, then Paris. Then you go on to Lyon and … Hang on. Pauline, you're not cruising up and down the Rhine, you're going up and down the Rhône instead." But what's really worrying is that we're still not sure that if we hadn't told her, she would have known any different. But the thought of Mam ordering drinks while speaking German in a Welsh accent to a French waiter was too much like *'Allo 'Allo* to let happen. Unless I could have been there to watch, of course. But the phrase book was not all in vain – even now, whenever anyone does or says something a little bit out of the ordinary in the shop, Mam says "Zach T" – it means "Easy, tiger!". But I think it's the only phrase she can remember, and only because it sounds like Zack's name.

Now we decided that the best thing to do was for Geraint to collect Mam from her friends', Jan and Mike Bull's, place in Basingstoke once she had returned to the UK, and I was not planning to go up so Geraint could break the news to her slowly and gently over the course of the journey. However that slow drip of information strategy turned to shit when Mam phoned me to confirm the collection arrangements and asked if I was coming up too, and when I said no she

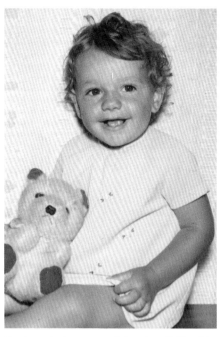 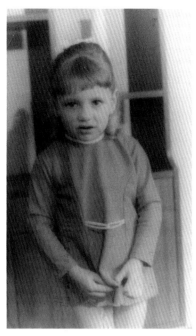

Sooty, what are you doing here? Hard to believe I was so angelic. Me, aged one.

Me aged three, no longer cherubic and my hair needs more attention.

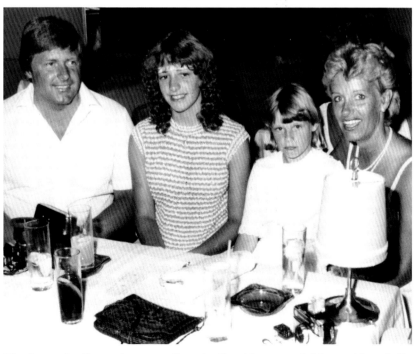

The James family getting away from it all, with me aged 16 now (from left): Dad, me, Kath and Mam.

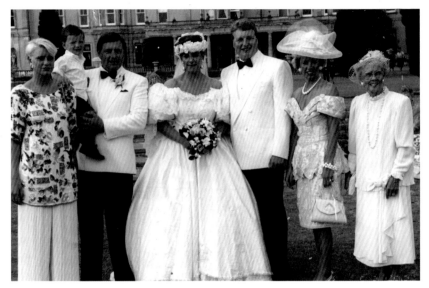

Our wedding day (from left): Kath, Zack and Dad, me and Geraint, Mam and Peggy, my nan. (Picture: Mark Cleghorn Photography)

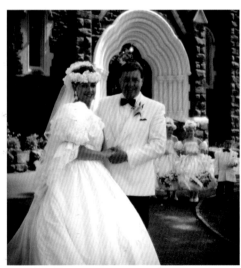

Dad and me on my wedding day outside St Mary's RC Church, Merthyr. (Picture: Mark Cleghorn Photography)

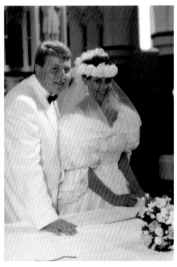

Geraint and I sign the register at St Mary's RC Church, Merthyr. (Picture: Mark Cleghorn Photography)

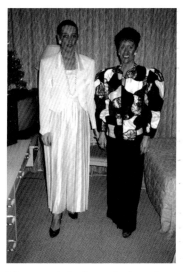

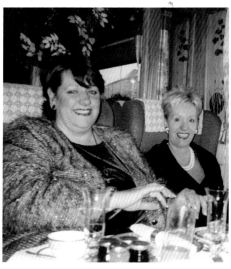

Mam and I channel American football and Dynasty in these outfits. Dig the crazy shoulder pads and hair.

Me at my largest, as Mam and I travel on the Venice-Simplon Orient Express.

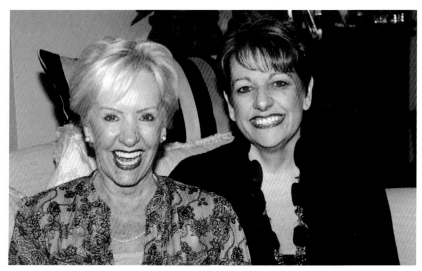

Mam has been a tower of strength throughout, and I often think that the madhouse that is her hairdressing business has kept me sane. (Picture: Judith Cooke Photography)

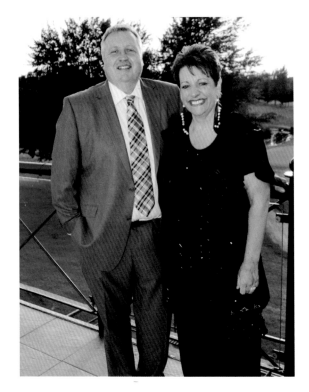

Geraint and I at Amy's wedding reception, just 24 hours after my first chemotherapy session. (Picture: Judith Cooke Photography)

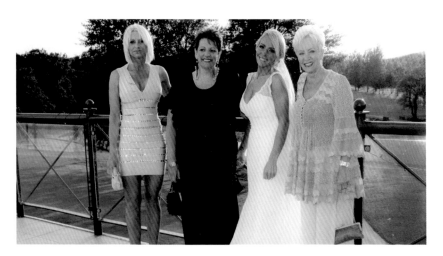

A family affair (from left): my sister Kath, me, the blushing bride Amy and Mam at Amy's wedding reception. (Picture: Judith Cooke Photography)

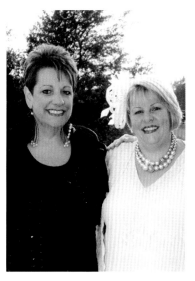

My surrogate elder sister Avalon and I. (Picture: Judith Cooke Photography)

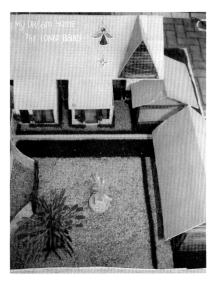

A model of our dream home for a BBC programme. (Picture: Charlotte Beattie)

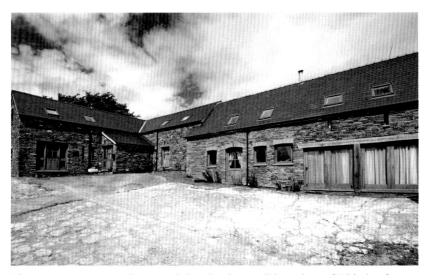

The programme never happened, but the dream did. A view of Rhiwlas from the old farmyard.

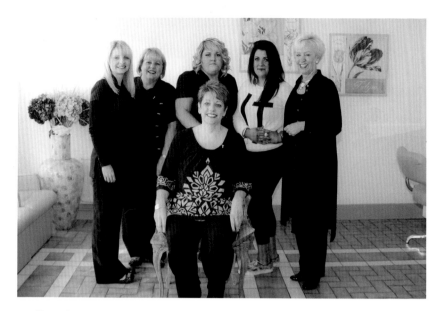

Pauline, the girls and me (from left): Jess Pulley, Avalon Thomas, me, Tarryn James, Kate James and Mam. It's never this formal usually – and Mam never lets them stand around!

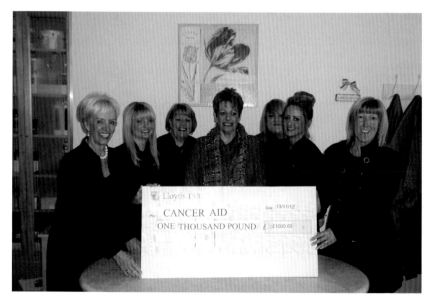

Mam's shop has done lots of fundraising for Cancer Aid Merthyr Tydfil (from left): Mam, Jess, Avalon, me, Tarryn, Zowie Griffiths and Tracey Burke from Cancer Aid.

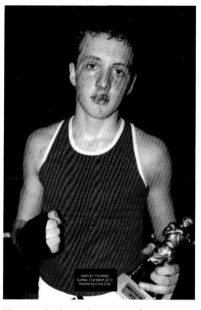

Harvey is the only one so far to get into the Thomas family business.

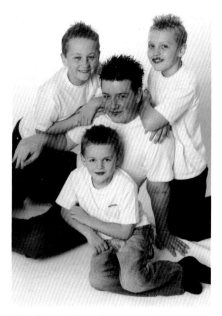

The boys (from left): Harrison, Zack and Harvey, with Roddy in front. (Picture: Photocolour Wales Ltd)

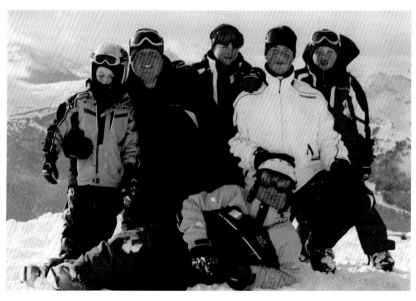

Out in Whistler, 2005 (kneeling, from left): Roddy, Geraint, Harrison, Zack and Harvey, with ski instructor Peter (lying in front).

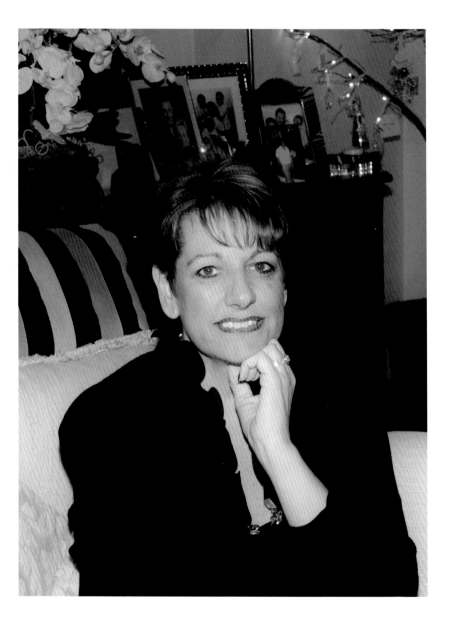

Glamming up for a photoshoot for the cover of this book, in the sitting room at Rhiwlas. (Picture: Judith Cooke Photography)

asked how things were. What do I do, what shall I say? Lying was out of the question, so I decided to go for the vague, buck-passing answer: "The results weren't quite as good as we'd hoped. Geraint will tell you about it when he picks you up."

As soon as Geraint, who had spent the whole journey up rehearsing what he should and shouldn't say, got to her friends' place in Basingstoke, Mam was in the car like a rat up a drainpipe, saying: "What's the news, what's happening?" So Geraint told her what the consultant had told us, and ended by saying that I was going to have chemotherapy. Mam brightened up at this – action was being taken so things could be fixed, and when he dropped her off Mam seemed in a pretty positive frame of mind.

Soon afterwards though, the phone rang in Brecon and it was Mam, going all Spanish Inquisition on me. "Annmarie, there's a message for you on my phone from the Royal Glamorgan Hospital. It says 'can you come in tomorrow?' You can listen to it if you want," and she played me the answerphone message. Basically it was asking me to contact Urology as soon as possible. I knew at once that it was to make arrangements for the operation to fit a stent. But that was the only hiccup in breaking the news to Mam.

I rang on the Monday morning, as soon as Urology could take my call, and took a bollocking from a very irate – and justifiably so – receptionist-cum-admin-istrator. We'd moved house and changed our numbers and not updated the records so we were pretty un-contactable. However, I had given them Mam's number as an emergency contact number so after they'd tried everything else except carrier pigeon, they decided to ring her. Of course she was bobbing up and down on the Rhône at this time, but at least she had an answerphone.

Anyway, the upshot of the call was that they wanted me in to do the procedure on Tuesday morning, so I had to come into the Royal Glamorgan in Llantrisant on Monday evening so I'd be there and ready and prepped for the op. When I arrived, I found they'd put me in a six-bed ward. Opposite me was an old lady who must have been in her 90s, who had obviously been in for a few days. As I was unpacking my bag, a nurse walked in and went over to her bed and asked: "Are these yours? I found them on the shelf in the toilet." I looked round, hoping against hope that the nurse was holding a pair of reading glasses – but no, just as I feared it was a set of extremely unattractive false teeth. I looked at Geraint and hissed: "Get me out of here!" If I'd gone into the loo and found false teeth on the shelf, I think I'd have dropped dead.

Two beds along was another woman who'd been in for a few weeks, but so far they couldn't diagnose what was wrong with her. In the bed next to mine was a young girl in her mid 20s who turned out to be something of a moaner. She was in agony, she said, and kept asking for painkillers. A male nurse came in and told her that he could only give her tablets to swallow now, and at that moment her parents came in and she burst into tears, saying "I can't swallow anything". Five minutes earlier she had been eating a large cooked dinner! The parents made a huge fuss of her and were looking daggers at the poor nurse. I caught Geraint's eye again: "Take me home or I swear I'll kill her!"

I was supposed to wait for the anaesthetist, but an hour in the ward had quite tired me out, so we went and told the nurse that we'd be popping off now, and would be back the following morning at 7am. "You can't do that, you may not have a bed in the morning," said the ward sister. "I'll take my chances," I said.

After all, who else was going to take it and stay there?

The following morning, I was back at Royal Glamorgan before 7am, just over 12 hours after I'd left there. The same ward sister I'd crossed swords with the night before was on duty still, and though she was a bit stroppy I was soon booked in (I mean "clerked in" – it isn't a hotel, you know); I suppose she's used to people listening to her and isn't ready for those of us with more independent minds.

We were sent to the waiting room to kill some time before being called, and I was reading my book while Geraint was getting to grips with the latest instalment of "why this country isn't what it used to be" from the *Daily Mail,* and then a couple walked in. The woman seemed OK, but was quite quiet; the husband was more your Valleys Boy bodybuilder type, with loads of tattoos and even more attitude. He walked in like The Terminator, kitted out in typical weightlifter mode – shorts, vest and flip-flops (all that was missing were the sunglasses) – to show off his abs, pecs, bi's, tri's, lats, glutes and any other abbreviated body parts you could think of. I wasn't sure if it was his wife or him who was the patient, but he did seem to be suffering from verbal diarrhoea. He also had a lisp.

It turned out that he was the patient, because we had a drama about "nil by mouth". He wasn't supposed to eat for 12 hours before coming in, "but I 'ad to 'ave this Challenge, see, 'cos I'm like, in training, see? And now, he announced, he was "'Ank Marvin" I didn't have a clue what he meant, but Geraint told me that he'd probably eaten a big meal far later than he should have done the night before and was complaining about being hungry because he was some sort of gym bunny. So it sort of made sense when the nurse told him that he was in theatre at 5 and therefore could not have anything substantial. Arnie was not impressed. "I'm

'Ank Marvin," he said. "'Ow the fucking hell am I going to last until 5 o'clock?" Then he started smoking a cigarette "to suppress my appetite, see" but the nurse came back to tell him that she, and the Local Health Board, would appreciate it if he did not smoke within the hospital buildings, which led to more moaning from the muscled one. I think that the nurse could tell he was one of the "If I make things really awkward people will give in to me just to shut me up" school of thought, and decided to offer him an olive branch. Or more accurately, a piece of toast. But he wasn't having any of that.

Sadly, before we got to find out whether Arnie would get his meal, or even beans on his toast, I was moved up on to the ward but, as I was being transported, I passed two nurses talking about the bodybuilder, and one said to the other: "If he keeps that up much longer, we'll move him to the side room." D'oh, which is exactly what he wants. It's a sad state of affairs when you have to give in to bullying, but I felt for the staff. What was the right thing to do? Keep him where he was because that was where he was supposed to be, but expose the rest of the patients to his moaning, whining and smoking? Or give into him, because even if it did make him feel better it would also do wonders for all the other poor souls who no longer had to listen to him? Tough call.

All this drama took my mind off the procedure I was actually in for, but a visit from the anaesthetist soon changed that. Because of the pain in my back, he said an epidural would be out of the question and I would have to undergo a general anaesthetic. Not my first choice – not even my last actually – but the time for quibbling seemed to have come and gone. We just had to get on with it and make the best of things. The consultant urologist operating on me was David Jones, a medic of the old school. You may recall that he was the surgeon who told me when I was diagnosed that had I left it three months before coming in, I'd have been dead. I saw the funny side of that then – I'm not sure if all his patients would, but he seemed to be able to judge who would respond best to being teased and who would do better with reassurance. But I think humour was his default position: you could tell David liked to banter with his patients – or at least he did with me – and I certainly appreciated that as it helped put me at ease. He told me that my Christmas present for this year would be a new stent – I said he could have a kiss if he was lucky, but more likely he'd be having the old one back!

My only medical concern then was the old BP – would my blood pressure be too high? I'd always seemed to suffer from "white coat syndrome" where regardless of how slowly it had been pumping up to that point, as soon as you showed me a BP monitor or a nurse it went straight through the roof. But the anaesthetist and David were both happy, so in I went. Before the operation, David told me that he was actually looking to put in two stents, even though I only needed one. I think that this was probably the better approach because, as it turned out, he couldn't get the left-hand side one in so I had to make do with just the one, on my right-hand side. All in all, it was a good day – despite the waiting room theatricals. I'd had a stent fitted and I'd undergone surgery with general anaesthetic without suffering any side-effects.

But a bigger problem had to be faced too. The last thing Geraint and I wanted to do was to tell the boys. We'd kept things on a need-to-know basis for a long time, with only Zack completely in the picture. But now, because we didn't know for sure how the treatment would affect me, we felt it was better that they knew what was going on, so they would understand why I might possibly be feeling so ill. We told them the night before I went in to begin my first chemotherapy treatment. They were very upset, naturally, but in a day or so they seemed to have bounced back to normal.

Looking back on things now, I realise that things could have been so much worse after I discovered that the cancer was back. Not so much from a medical point of view, because we quickly did all the things that needed to be done, but from the effect the news might have had on Mam. Really, I can't get over how strong she's been all the way through with me, just like she was with Dad. To be honest, I thought that having gone through it once, it would hit her harder second time around and she would find it difficult to cope, but not a bit of it.

One change it has brought out in her is her attitude to the medical "emergencies" of others. In the shop, she hasn't got any patience with the customers who come in with the usual niggles and moans, as every medical condition is measured (unfairly or not) against mine. Colds and sprains are given short shrift; nothing less than full amputation at the neck is a sufficient reason to gripe now: "You've just got to get on with it, haven't you? Annmarie, now she's got cancer, but look at her – she's a rock." Mam doesn't ask how I am – she knows I won't give her an honest answer if I'm not feeling too clever – and she says "I know you'll be fine." But I think she's afraid that one day she'll ask how I'm feeling and I'll tell her the truth.

Most of the time, I'm good and tell myself and everyone else that I'm going to be fine, but I do occasionally get black days. One day I'd been to Velindre to give blood and I was feeling really low, so when I came home I just went up to lie on the bed. I was feeling really rough and totally out of sorts, and I lost it a bit so I lay there crying. In walked Mam, and she'd never really seen me crying before and certainly not because I didn't feel well. The sight and sound of me pushed her over the edge a bit and she got hysterical and had to go home, and when she got back she cried her eyes out all over again. But it's good that she's getting support too – Nan is spiritual and so is Avalon, both my and Mam's best friend (and longest employee at the shop too) and they have both been telling her that "Annmarie is strong, and she's going to come through the other side of it."

So, to some extent, this means that Mam can treat me exactly the same as before – but there are downsides to that. Now Mam is obsessed by weight, she always has been. And for the last few decades, that has meant being obsessed with my weight. I've always been well covered, as they say in Merthyr, but I wasn't that heavy at school and I was very fit almost naturally. Mam watches her weight, and my sister is a fitness nut, but I suppose I have tended to favour and follow my dad's side of the family, the ones who eat and drink well but not always wisely. But I do recall being taken to Weight Watchers at the age of 18, and being told to lose two stone. That was really lost on me and when she used to watch me getting something from the kitchen, or putting another potato on my plate, she'd say, "Do you really need that?"

Once I got married though and had four boys, that was when I really started to put on the pounds. I loved to cook for Geraint, and he loved to eat what I cooked for him so we both gained weight. There was no guilt about eating food, so we both did. Then when I became ill and started to lose weight, Mam was on my case wanting to know if I was trying to diet – "Can you eat that? Are you allowed that" – even now that I have cancer. I mean, are you being serious, Mam? In the last month or so, I've shed a couple of stone and Mam asked me what I weighed. I told her: "13st 12lbs." "How much have you lost then?" said Mam. I said I didn't know, and so she continued: "Are you planning to lose any more?" Meanwhile I'm thinking to myself: "This is ridiculous. She can't seem to grasp that I may have changed my diet, but I'm not dieting." For the record and for Mam, to date I've lost 15st in 18 months.

But at least it meant she was treating me normally. And once the chemo started in earnest, I was going to need all the normality I could get.

# Chapter Ten

## Chemotherapy Doesn't Have to Ruin Your Life

Gratitude is the attitude
*Annmarie James-Thomas*

It's funny the sort of things that go through your mind when you are given bad news. The first thought that went through my head after I realised that I was going to have to undergo some form of chemotherapy wasn't about the long-term chances of success or even the possibilities of hair loss (it's quite likely, I suppose, that I'd done so much research into my cancer by this stage that I already knew the answers to those and a host of other questions, so I didn't feel the need to ask). No, my questions were all to do with a wedding I was supposed to be going to the day after my first chemo. How would I feel then, given that I was having the chemo just 24 hours before? "You'll feel OK on the Friday straight after you've had it," I was told, "but by Saturday it will really start to hit home. It'll feel like you've been hit by a 10-ton truck."

I was absolutely devastated – the bride was Amy, the daughter of Avalon, my mam's and my best friend. Amy was a bridesmaid at my wedding and, naturally, I wanted to be there for her on her big day. We'd been invited to go to Italy with them and not been able to go because of the cancer, but to miss the wedding party too was just too much to think about. I broke the news to Avalon, and she was just lovely about it. "Don't say you're definitely not coming now," she said. "See how you feel. Let's play it by ear. Come if you're up to it; and if you don't feel well enough, please don't worry but just get yourself some rest and recharge."

So I wasn't in the best frame of mind when I went to Nevill Hall Hospital in Abergavenny for my first treatment – and it wasn't just the thought of missing the wedding. Don't forget, the way that the chemo sapped the strength of my father is probably the strongest memory I have of his cancer, and I had done everything I could to avoid that happening to me. And yet here I was, despite my best efforts and those of a whole array of nurses, radiographers, doctors and surgeons, sitting in the hospital and waiting to begin treatment. Even now, though, I had opted for the less toxic carboplatin treatment rather than the stronger, but more side-effect ridden, paclitaxel.

Some people reading this from outside South Wales may be confused by the comparatively large number of hospitals I have been going to for treatment, so a quick explanation is in order. When I lived in Merthyr, I was in the catchment area for the Cwm Taf Health Board, and the hospitals here included Prince Charles Hospital (which is actually in Merthyr) and the Royal Glamorgan Hospital (in Llantrisant). Depending on what your medical condition is and the surgeons or specialists involved, you may be treated at one, the other or both of these. In addition to the cancer specialists at these hospitals, and also at the Cardiff and Vale University Health Board (which is served by the University of Wales Hospital and University Hospital Llandough among others), most of Wales' cancer treatment and expertise is offered by the Velindre NHS Trust, which is located in the Cardiff suburb of Whitchurch. When I moved to Brecon, I moved into the Aneurin Bevan Local Health Board area, which is served by, among others, the Royal Gwent Hospital in Newport and Nevill Hall Hospital. Now Prince Charles Hospital is just as close in terms of distance and probably easier to drive to than, Nevill Hall, but because I live in Brecon, I had to go to Nevill Hall for my treatment, even though my support network is all based near Merthyr and I tend to be there most of the time anyway.

And that was how I found myself in a small waiting room at Nevill Hall. I've already told you how I suffer from claustrophobia – remember my terrors about the enclosed MRI scanner? – and so I asked the nurses if it would be possible to be seated as near to the door as they could manage, to minimise any tension I might begin to feel. The nurses must have sensed my nervousness because nothing was too much trouble and they moved me into a quiet side room which just had one bloke in it. Instead of a door, it was curtained off from the main waiting room – so I felt absolutely fine and not in the least bit penned in. Then a nurse came to put a line into my hand, which was quite difficult as I don't have very prominent veins at the best of times. The needle went in and she flushed it with a saline solution, and then began to take my blood pressure. Just as she did I started to feel very dizzy, so bad that I asked if the nurse could open the window. My blood pressure was falling through the floor. The chemotherapy nurse came over and said that there was no way they could start to administer the chemo if that was my reaction after only the saline drip was passed through the line. The best option was to hook me up to a heart monitor for an hour and see what was happening.

Now the books they give you to read up about the chemotherapy treatment you will be having talk about the possible side-effects, and say that you may be given some tablets to help minimise the effects of sickness. But I had decided that, initially at least, I certainly wouldn't be taking any anti-sickness pills or steroids, as I didn't want any false sense of well-being. I wanted to know exactly what my body was telling me. And initially, it looked like my body was telling me: "Get me out of here!"

So there I was, about to start a treatment I didn't want but needed, and then it seemed that I couldn't have it after all because my blood pressure was too low. It couldn't get any worse, could it? Well actually, yes it could, and it did. Remember the man in the corner? I hadn't – but then he piped up. He was having chemo too, he said, and in fact he was a chemotherapy veteran – he'd had "300 chemos" in his time, apparently. But that wasn't enough; the man, who was dressed as if he might be some sort of farmer, was also an expert on his family's cancer care too, as I discovered only too quickly. "My wife had cancer," he said, "and the first time she had chemotherapy her heart stopped and they had to resuscitate her." Great, just what I wanted to hear, I thought.

The nurse came back to ask me a few questions just to eliminate any variables. The first question was whether or not I was diabetic? (No, I'm not.) "I'm diabetic," said my new best friend from the corner of the room. Anything I had or didn't have, he'd had first – and worse – or if he hadn't then his wife had. And at that moment, the curtains twitched. Thank God, I said to myself, it's someone coming to rescue me, or at least pump me full of mind-numbing drugs. But no, it was the wife about whom I had heard so much (far more than I needed to, and much more than I wanted to), and he started the story once again of how she'd nearly died, only this time I got added information from the almost-late-and-lamented missus. "I didn't know anything about it but they nearly lost me," she said. Truly, waiting for my blood pressure to rise was the longest hour I have ever spent in my life, and certainly the most painful.

But rise it did, and soon I was hooked up to a carboplatin line, and Elvis was in the building. I felt fine, a lot better than I had when I was listening to that twerp (in fairness, I think he was just trying to be nice and make conversation; but whereas David Jones, my Urology surgeon, appeared to be able to read exactly what people wanted to hear, that vital skill had passed my room-mate by). But as I relaxed I was able to look through the gap in the curtain, which had not been fully closed, and see who was in the main – though incredibly small – room. I could see a man and his wife (she was the patient) and another man in his late 50s who was having chemotherapy. I don't know what it is about chemotherapy but it seems to make men more garrulous, because for the three hours I was there, his was the only voice I could hear. I'm not sure who he was talking to; it might have been the other people in the waiting room, or the nurses – he might even have been talking to himself, but whoever his audience was he didn't stop. And what a story he had to tell (some details have been changed to protect the guilty!).

It seemed this man worked in a large superstore in the Heads of the Valleys area, but only on the night shift. But he was coining it – in fact he'd earned so much there that he'd bought himself a Ferrari sports car. Now how he'd got into shelf stacking wasn't really clear because he had been a women's hairdresser in one of the towns along the A465 Heads of the Valleys road (my ears pricked up at that one, but I didn't hear anything to give me a clue as to who he was). Why he'd given up the cut-and-thrust of the cut-and-blow-dry I couldn't tell because his customers loved him – he couldn't do enough for them. Why, one Christmas morning he opened the shop and did 12 perms before going home to stuff his bird and scrub his sprouts.

How I didn't laugh, I just don't know. Others were not so lucky – the guy who was in the room with his wife started to lose it. He started to make occasional eye contact with me and once he saw we were on the same page as far as the Valleys' Vidal Sassoon was concerned he began to roll his eyes as the tall tales just kept on coming. He didn't exactly stuff a handkerchief in his mouth but if he hadn't excused himself from the room then that would have been the next step. But as he went down the corridor, you could hear him laughing his socks off, and then apologising to the nurse, saying: "I'm sorry, but we just couldn't help ourselves." The nurses said that was OK, because they were used to it. Last month apparently, the man had brought in a picture he was showing round to all the nurses, saying that it was his son and asking if they'd like to go out on a date with him – but it was obvious the picture had been cut from a magazine and stuck onto a piece of card. "But don't worry about him," they said. "There's another bloke who comes in here who's ten times worse."

So that was my first chemotherapy session. Far more entertaining than I expected it to be and, once my blood pressure got out of the basement, far less uncomfortable too. I didn't die on the gurney and I didn't have any immediate reactions. Now all I had to do was wait for the side-effects. I was pretty sure that I wouldn't be there at my best friend's daughter's wedding to see Amy walk down the aisle.

And it looked as if the doctors might be right. On

the Friday, I felt just like the doctors said I would – absolutely fine. Apart from lying down for an hour while they trickled the carboplatin into me, it was just a normal day at the office. Of course I knew that the next day I was going to feel horrible, so I decided to just make the most of it and enjoy the calm before the storm. On Saturday morning, I woke up at the usual time, feeling completely ... normal. But it was obviously going to hit me soon – the doctors had said so. An hour passed, and nothing had happened. At this point, I had a couple of options: I could either sit around waiting for the tiredness to spread over me and be paralysed, or I could be me. I decided to be me, and jumped in the car and tore straight up to Merthyr for some of what Geraint calls "Princess Time". One of the great advantages of having a mother who is a hairdresser is that you never have to make an appointment. Meanwhile, I was waiting for the tiredness to kick in – and still it didn't. Straight after my hair appointment, I went shopping for something to wear to the wedding, went home and changed. All day I was waiting for something to happen, some change in the way I felt to tell me that the chemo was taking effect, but nothing came. In fact, it wasn't until the following Wednesday that the side-effects came. I was so pleased that I'd been able to be there for my friend's day – and in time I became pleased that a pattern had established itself, so that I knew how many days' grace I had after chemo before I started to feel under the weather.

It wasn't even as if we took it easy either – we actually left the wedding at about 11.30pm, having been seated on a table with my sister and her husband among others. Also sitting there was a friend of Avalon's who is a teacher at Bishop Hedley, and her husband, a barrister. Geraint went to the bar to get a round of drinks, and while he was bringing them back we heard a loud POP as he stepped on a foil-wrapped packet of butter, the contents of which shot across the room and hit the barrister full in the face, as well as making a nice greasy mark on his suit jacket. That seemed to set the tone for the day. I tried to dance with John, the bride's father, but my legs were killing me and I knew it was time to go when I nearly fell over, and began to laugh so hard that I started to wet myself. "I'm peeing myself," I told him. I'm sure he thought I just meant I was laughing hard – but I didn't, and a trickle of urine really did run down my leg!

Three weeks later I was sitting down ready for my second cycle of carboplatin, this time at the Macmillan Suite in Prince Charles Hospital (I'd swapped my treatment location – everyone was only too happy to help me fit in). Things seemed far less stressful and rushed at Prince Charles than at Nevill Hall – the nurses were lovely and everything was somehow calmer. There were two other women in for chemotherapy when I was there: a curly-permed woman in her 70s who was on her own and said she lived in the Rhondda, and a younger woman from Pontypridd, who had come in with her husband (who hadn't yet joined us). I sat down with Geraint and looked across at the older woman, who had a book. "What are you reading?" I asked. Then I saw the cover photograph of an expensively patterned silver silk tie. "*50 Shades of Grey*," she said, not remotely embarrassed. She was really enjoying the book – she'd been there, done that and got the mink-lined handcuffs and flogger, as it were!

The woman introduced herself as Moira, and she turned out to be a very chatty person. She asked what sort of treatment I was having and told me that she was going for the combined carboplatin-paclitaxel regimen.

I said that I'd considered the combined course but ultimately decided against it. "Why's that then?" she said. "I'd rather not say," was my response, because I didn't want to go into the fact that I'd done research and thought the side effects sounded horrendous. "Ooooh," the woman said. The other woman was very quiet – almost too quiet. She was acting a bit like they tell you to act if there is a comedian on stage in a club, and the last thing you want to do is anything that draws attention to yourself. But too late; Moira saw the woman and turned her attention from me to her. "I ordered a wig just like that," she said to the younger woman. "It's being delivered next week." I didn't realise she was wearing a wig; hang on, I didn't realise they were both wearing wigs! "They're expensive," she continued, looking more closely at the younger woman's 'syrup'. "Is it real hair?" No, the younger one replied. "They cost about £400."

By now, the younger woman was starting to worry about her husband, who still hadn't joined us after parking their car. "Don't worry about him," I said. "He's probably in the Gurnos Club nursing a pint before going to the bookies' to put a bet on." She carried on fretting so Geraint volunteered to go and find him, as the woman said their car was in the car park. "What sort of car is it?" Geraint asked. "A blue one," was the reply. Five minutes later, Geraint was back: no sign of the man in the side car park. "No, he wouldn't be," said the woman. "He went to the main car park." Geraint was about to go again when the man appeared. "Thank God for that," I said. "Your wife thought you were dead. We've sent the police out looking for you."

So another chemo, another funny story. And that was pretty much how it went. Every session I met someone new with something to say, and I had a lot of laughs. And that's important – we may be ill, but we don't have to act like we are, at least not all of the time. In my case, I was definitely getting more than enough emotional sustenance and support from my family and close friends, and also by drawing all the humour I could from the situation I found myself in. But what about my physical well-being? How was I responding to the treatment?

The first three cycles of chemotherapy – three weeks apart – went really well I felt, almost like clockwork. I had the chemo on the Friday, and after the first scary session when my blood pressure collapsed, there were no particular scares or side-effects at all. I would be fine over the weekend, but by about Tuesday I'd start to get diarrhoea, and feel really tired as the effects of the chemo kicked in. But by the Friday I'd feel fine again. I was only suffering for three days out of 21, which I reckoned was pretty good, so I reckoned I'd chosen the right course of chemo to follow. The fourth session was different though, as I started to feel ill on the Monday, but I was prepared for this. I had been told that the more chemos I had, the more the chemicals would accumulate in my body and take longer to clear, so I was sort of "topping up" and the sickness was coming sooner as a result. But that wasn't anything I couldn't deal with.

But what about the one side-effect that I had been hoping for? Did the chemo do anything to fix my sense of taste and smell? Not in the slightest. Despite the chemo I was still struggling with both tastes and smells. One day I popped into the shop and Avalon came to give me a kiss on the cheek. The smell of her perfume was just so powerful that I couldn't help myself. "You're absolutely buzzing," I told her. Even the mildest of things can set me off, so more intense smells are like electric shocks to my system.

The food I could eat on the Hippocrates diet is pretty bland, to say the least, but even that was too spicy and strong for me. So in a bid to eat something, I took myself off that diet and instead tried more normal foods instead for variety. I eat very little and avoid meats wherever possible, but I do have a little scrambled egg on occasion. I've done my best not to let my aversion to food smells and tastes get in the way of family life, and the first time we went out for a meal after my chemo started, I ordered a beef dinner. It was absolutely delicious and though I couldn't eat it all, I loved what I did manage (and Geraint got to finish the food I had left on my plate!). We have been to a couple of nice places since then – The Inn at Penallt (a gastropub) and the Felinfach Griffin Inn – and we've had a really good time. But when you're paying good money for a main course that you cannot eat, and not because there's anything wrong with it either, then it does sort of put a dampener on things. It's not just main courses either: one weekend we went out and I fancied some flapjacks and panna cotta, but when the sweet arrived, I could only manage two mouthfuls before I had to leave the room. And it's always a bit awkward when waiters come back and see I've left so much on the plate and ask if anything was wrong with the food. I don't know if they believe me when I say: "It's not you; it's me." I mean, does anyone? I tell them that I'd eaten more than I'd realised before coming out, and just couldn't finish my lovely meal.

And that's the truth, sort of. The food is lovely, but I'm ill. I shouldn't be scared to say: "I'm not well, so could I have a smaller portion please?" But I don't want to do that – it's not the sort of attention people like to draw to themselves. Geraint does his bit to make the waiters feel more comfortable though. When we went to The Bear, he wanted chicken pie but actually ordered a cheese sandwich because he knew he would be finishing my meal.

But even when you do ask for smaller portions it doesn't always work out. During the summer, I went out for lunch with the Cricket Wives (or should I say Cricket Widows!) Basically, all our sons play for the local cricket club, and we meet up most weekends for games during the summer, doing the teas or watching the game through those most wonderful of binoculars (the bottom of a glass of wine). From time to time we go out to lunch, and this time we went to Alfred's Bistro in Pontypridd. I ordered a salad and I fancied scallops, which was on the menu as a starter, so I asked if I could have that as my main course, as I knew three scallops would fill me. But the waitress brought me five – and in the end I could only eat two. Chefs are funny creatures – but they don't like to disappoint, and I think that they gave me more because they thought it would please me, and if my appetite had been better it certainly would have done, but when I saw the plate with five on it, I knew I was buggered.

And there's the thing; you don't want to create a fuss, but anything you say is effectively going to do just that, so I sometimes think it's easier if I just don't go out at all.

But even if I'm having problems nourishing my body, healing my spirit is far easier to do as I'm getting plenty of "the best medicine". And for that, I don't need to visit any hospitals or clinics.

# Chapter Eleven

## Welsh Penicillin from the Soup Kitchen

A good laugh and a long sleep are the best cures in the
doctor's book
***Irish proverb***

Everyone has heard of "Jewish penicillin", which is
often used when people talk about chicken soup,
especially the Jewish sort made not only with chicken
but also egg noodles or fine spaghetti. It's a bit of an
old wives' tale, but it's traditionally seen not only as a
food but also as a pick-me-up and cure-all for colds,
flu and stomach problems. Less well known but just as
effective is Welsh penicillin, the particular sense of fun
and laughter that you find in people from the
principality. There are different recipes, I'm sure, with
North Walian and West Walian flavours being fairly
distinctive. But it's the South Wales flavour I know
best, and that's certainly the one for me. And the best
soup kitchen in Wales is found on Merthyr's Brecon
Road. But it's not very well-known, except by its
customers, as it is cunningly disguised as a ladies'
hairdresser's.

Pauline's really is a place of laughter, where I'm
sure people come to be entertained just as much as
groomed, and where you are made to feel part of a big
family. Women come there from across South Wales
to get their hairdos, and though the stylists there are

very, very good, it can't just be that that keeps people coming back, even when they move from town. Both Jeremy's aunts go there, and his cousins – that's all his immediate female family in Merthyr – and they have been regulars there for years. It's a Merthyr institution – and that's probably the right word to use for it. Because although you don't have to be mad to work there, it certainly helps if you are.

I sometimes wonder how Mam does it – she's a very bright lady. But then she's often just as crazy as the others. I told Jeremy he had to visit the shop to get an idea of what it was like, because it is almost indescribable. A lot of the women who go there to have their hair done are business people and professionals, with more than a few doctors and teachers, and I think that they all go to Pauline's for the same reason: it's the fun factor. And more than one has told Mam that it's a shame you can't get the therapy you get there from the NHS as a prescription drug.

Pauline's has been at Brecon Road for the past 30 years – in fact it's never been anywhere else, as it was the first business Mam opened when I was just 11. Like I said, Mam was always a bright girl – she passed her 11-plus and then went to the County Grammar School in Merthyr and did her exams. Then she trained as a hairdresser and worked at a couple of the town's better-known salons. I don't know if she was becoming restless, or was looking for a new challenge, but whatever it was she needed more than she was getting just cutting and styling hair for other people. I'm not sure Dad was the driving force behind her setting up the business, but he was certainly the one who saw the opportunity and the gap in the market. One day he came home from work and said: "I've seen a shop for sale on the Brecon Road. It's already a hairdresser's."

It was too, run by a bloke, but he was looking to get out of the business, so Mam went along and had a look, made an offer and moved in. As part of the asking price she got fixtures and fittings, as well as goodwill – and she also got Avalon.

Avalon has been my mam's – and my – best friend for years, and really it's hard to think of a time when she hasn't been in our life. She had been working at the shop for two years before Mam bought it, and she sort of came with the furniture. And, apart from breaks to have her children, Amy and Jonathan, she's never been away. I often say she's like my sister, but that's a lie – she's far more than that. She's the big sister I never had, and probably always needed. She and I were always great together but it wasn't until I was 18 or 19 that the age gap between us seemed to disappear and we became very close. It's funny but people do really think we are sisters, and physically we certainly are alike – we have the same olive skin and dark eyes. Our families are close, her daughter Amy was one of my bridesmaids and we have gone on holidays together. Before I became ill, most Thursdays Mam, Avalon and I would have a girls' film night; we'd go from the shop at closing time, get something to eat and then pop down to the Vue multiscreen cinema in Merthyr to catch the latest blockbuster or comedy. It trailed off for me a bit when I became ill, though Mam and Avalon continue to go. I know that if I need something I can just pick up the phone and ring Avalon, and if she can do it for me then she will – and she knows I'd do the same for her. She is a star.

I know that's true because of the huge part she's played in both my and my dad's cancer, supporting us and – just as important – supporting Mam and propping her up when she needed it. Avalon, Mam, Dad and I are all "glass half full" people, who try to find the silver lining inside every cloud and can always be counted on to spin things positively; Alastair Campbell has got nothing on us! By comparison, Kath is far more realistic and tends to see things as they are, and that's good – but sometimes you need that sense of optimism otherwise you'd just give up, put your head under the blanket and not bother to get up in the morning.

When I broke the news of my cancer to her, she was very good and tried to be strong about things – though I could tell she was really upset. After we'd talked she went back home and bawled like a basket case; she was so beside herself that she just had to let it out. She told me about it a few days later though, but only when she thought I'd be able to handle the thought of her being weak. She sees things from her friends' and family's point of view all the time – when I told her I had cancer she kept asking herself "Why is this happening to Annmarie?" She was in a terrible state and when she went to work the next day she broke down in tears (all the girls in the shop did too, when they heard – we really are all that close and just like a family). When I heard about that, I rang her in the evening and we talked; she was being very matter-of-fact and trying to keep from showing how upset she was. I had enough on my plate, was her way of thinking, and the last thing I needed was to be worried and upset about how she was.

That's the sort of girl Avalon is. But we're so close that I can tell what is going on inside, and she can do the same with me: we can read each other like books. She gets very excited about things, though she does her best to hide it. When she's emotional, you can tell because she takes a deep breath and talks and talks, it's like she's afraid to stop talking and let go. The first time she came up to the barn, she talked for ages, looked round and said how nice it was then went home and sobbed her heart out for an hour. She knew how much I'd wanted this and was so happy for us that we were living in our dream home. She felt so emotional being there and seeing all the work that we had put into it.

We've always had dramas, Avalon and I, on both sides over the years but we've been there for each other always. She's great with my mam too, and when she has wobbles it's good to know that Avalon is there to keep an eye on her, and help her along if she needs a hand to hold. Then I'll get a call in the evening telling me if something has happened. When we are together I can tell if Mam has been upset; we're very close like that and I can sense her moods. She only appears to be calm and unflappable on the surface, but she really isn't. And that's why it's good that Avalon is there. She really is a great person to have in your life. And that's why Pauline's is such a happy place to work, and to go for a hairdo.

But it's not just Avalon; all the girls are larger-than-life characters and they all bring something different to the party. Avalon is a lot like me, very spiritual and a bit earth-mother, in the best possible way. Jess is very good, very funny with a dry sense of humour, which you wouldn't think given that she also lectures in hairdressing at Merthyr College. Zowie, Tarryn and Tarryn's sister Kate are younger than the others, so the girls in the shop cover the whole age range (and Tarryn and Kate are family, they're my second cousins on my dad's side). Tarryn's claim to fame is that she's a human filing cabinet and card index. She knows everyone in Merthyr and how they are connected to everyone else, which is a great skill for a hairdresser to have: knowing who's who is just as important as how to cut the latest style.

111

I saw the healing powers of Pauline's at first hand after Dad died: it really was a godsend. The shop gave Mam's life a structure and a reason to get up in the morning, if ever she felt down in the dumps, and having to deal with the girls and the people who came in to be styled meant that she couldn't shut herself away for long. I don't think she's likely to retire now, even if she cuts her hours and works less. She did think about selling up and retiring at one time, so that she and Dad could spend their golden years together but then he was diagnosed, and that took her away from the day-to-day running of the business a lot. And after the cancer took him, it was Pauline's that helped her come to terms with things, as I honestly think her grief was so great that she would have killed herself after he died, good Catholic girl or not.

A month after my dad died, in the first week in December, we went to Lille for the Christmas markets. We had booked the trip before he had started to really decline, and Mam had decided she was going to stay in Wales with him. I realised that he wasn't likely to be with us by the time the trip came around, so Avalon and I talked about it and decided that we wouldn't take her name off the booking, just in case. And a week before we were due to go I told her that we still had a place for her. It was lovely just to be able to go off and see different scenery and have different conversations – there were no partners there and it was a bloody good laugh. Then after her return, as she felt stronger, she went back to work just before Christmas. As she said: "There's only so much shopping you can do." And though for a while she lived to work, whereas before she had only worked to live, it helped her get through the bad days, because even if her nights were dark and lonely, her days were full of life and laughter.

And there's plenty of laughter. It's almost as if

every day something different is happening there to brighten the day, like the day when Avalon broke the door. Now I wouldn't say that Avalon is a little rough, but Mam won't let her touch anything new, delicate or in any way breakable in the shop. It's not as if Avalon is heavy-handed but … OK, she really is heavy-handed. One morning there had been a rush on, and as Avalon had finished her client and popped the lady's head under the dryer, she took the opportunity to do a bit of sweeping up to clear the floor. Now Avalon's sweeping is the stuff of legend; if she's upstairs and brushing away, it sounds like she's got one of those industrial vacuum cleaners it's so noisy. So on this day she was whirling around like a Dervish; a bit of vigorous sweeping and she rapped the toughened glass door with the end of her sweeping brush. It's the sort of thing that happens all the time. Except this was Avalon. Crash! Toughened glass in pieces and a big hole where the door used to be. A quick phone call to the glaziers and in an hour or so the door was fixed. More importantly it added another story to the legend of Pauline's.

When Jeremy went there for a day, just to get a feel for the place, I don't think he was ready for what he discovered, even though he had been warned. But after he'd listened to the stories that came out as Pauline, Avalon, Jess, Zowie, Tarryn and Kate cut and washed the customers' hair, he said it was more like episodes of *Friends*, with each story having its own little title. Here are a few that he liked, because they are funny but also because they will give you more of an insight into the girls of Pauline's. And not surprisingly, a lot of them involve Avalon…

**The one where the kettle went all frothy coffee**

The girls keep the shop spotless during the working day, so the coffee cups that are given to the customers are ferried upstairs to be washed on a regular basis, because that's where the kitchen is. Mam and Avalon were up there rinsing out the cups, and one of them filled the bowl with Fairy Liquid. Now no one knows exactly what happened because neither Mam nor Avalon are prepared to accept responsibility for this one, but somehow Fairy Liquid got into the kettle – and not just a splash of it either. Anyway, the kettle – which was empty after having made a load of coffees – was refilled and set to boil and Mam and Avalon came downstairs. Soon, one of the other girls went upstairs to make more coffee only to find loads of bubbles pouring out of the kettle spout just like you'd see in a sitcom. She comes downstairs, yelling that something was happening to the kettle and it was foaming at the mouth, and the shop disintegrates into laughter. Now, though neither Mam nor Avalon owned up, an unwritten rule seems to have developed that if no one else is responsible, then Avalon gets the blame. This may be a little harsh because Mam doesn't tend to hold up her hands either …

**The one where the customer 'lost' her car keys**

Now Mam has a thing about car keys, about which more later, but her most irritating habit is picking up other people's keys. Mam's key ring is like a jailer's – keys for everything – and topped off with one of those clever little Tesco Clubcard fobs, and she tends to use the Tesco fob as a way of recognising her keys: if there's a fob, it's Mam's bunch.

One Friday, one of our regular customers – let's call her Joan (because her name *is* Joan) – parked outside the salon and came in but, as many of our customers do, left her bag in the car. When one of the girls came to start styling her hair, Joan put her keys on the shelf in front of the mirror and sat down. But after she'd finished, Joan could not find her keys. The girls looked all over the shop – under cushions, behind sofas – but nothing. Now, from time to time things get tidied up from the shelf in the course of the day – mainly the coffee cups – so the girls checked the kitchen as well. Not a bean. Directing the search and rescue operation was Mam, supervising everyone's areas of responsibility to ensure the keys didn't get missed, and getting everyone to check their bags just in case someone had picked up the key. In the end, Joan left, slightly peeved, after Mam called for a taxi to take her home; she had a spare set of keys at home and her son could bring her back down to collect the car. And that's what must have happened because on Saturday morning, the car had gone from outside the salon.

That day Mam ordered another search of the property – and yet again the girls found nothing. There was no sign of Joan's keys – a car key and house key with a Tesco Clubcard fob. Then on Monday, Mam asked me to get something from her handbag – one of those ones with 20 different pockets, zips and compartments. I couldn't find whatever it was she'd asked me to get so I started ferreting and came up with ... Joan's keys, zipped away in one of Mam's many pockets. Mam was very apologetic, of course, but said it could have happened to anyone, right?

**The one where Avalon went blind**

I've already told you about Avalon's prowess with the sweeping brush, but this one had to be seen to be believed. One day, she was sweeping up and put her brush down flat on the floor and turned away to pick up something. Then she turned back and stood on the head of the brush and the shaft came flying up and hit her bang in the face, just like one of those cartoons where Tom stands on a rake as he chases Jerry round the garden. Instinctively Avalon shut her eyes to prevent damage. Then she screamed: "Pauline, Annmarie. Come quick, I've gone blind!"

What had seemed funny as we watched from behind was suddenly real and serious, so we came running. Avalon was standing there, crying: "I can't see, I can't see!" And then Mam got to her and started laughing. "Avalon, you can't see because your eyes are closed!" She'd forgotten to open them again. So she did, and said: "That's better!"

### The one where Zowie gave the Pole a closer shave than he expected

This was one of those train-wreck moments where you can just see it happening, but you can't seem to do anything to stop it. Pauline's clientele is predominantly female, but the girls can cut men's hair too, and often do. On one occasion, Tarryn was cutting the hair of a Polish man, and after she'd finished cutting his hair, she asked if he'd like his moustache trimmed as well, and he said he did. Now Tarryn does not normally like to trim moustaches; it's just one of those phobia things, like the way some people are frightened of clowns or buttons. So she asked Zowie if she'd do the trimming for her.

Up Zowie stepped, and picked up the trimmers and started to remove the extra hair. But I don't know what happened, but for some reason she didn't put the guard on, so instead of just removing the stray longer hairs, the clipper went right down to the skin. We just stood (or, in my case, sat) there slightly shocked, and it almost happened in slow motion. Zowie realised what she'd done just as soon as it was too late to stop. But what could she do now? It wasn't as if she could leave the other half in place, was it?

As luck would have it, at this moment in time she was standing between the Pole and the mirror so he couldn't see exactly what had happened; So, staying where she was and blocking his view of his reflection, Zowie leaned across smartly and chopped off the other side. And that was it, done. But then I think she realised what had happened because she ran upstairs to hide! And that left poor Tarryn to ask the poor Pole who was now looking in the mirror, almost disbelieving and running his hand across his upper lip: "Is that all right?"

What could the poor man say? He muttered something which Tarryn took to mean "Absolutely marvellous", paid his money and left the shop. One of the girls watched him as he walked along the road, and started laughing as he stopped at every one of the nearby shops' plate glass windows, looking at his missing facial fuzz and shaking his head. Then he walked past a Polish shop at the end of the street; the shopkeeper was standing on the doorstep and as an animated conversation followed, accompanied by much gesticulating and pointing towards our shop; we could only guess what was being said but it didn't sound good. Now, every time he walks past the shop, Zowie starts to brick it, and we keep on telling her that one day he's going to come in.

**The one where Pauline's car keys didn't work**

Not every funny story happens at the shop. One day, Pauline was not in work, but had to do some banking so she drove from her home in Church Village to Pontypridd, and parked her car in the open-air car park in Taff Street, near to the bank. But when she came back, she couldn't remember exactly where she had parked it, so she walked around in vain looking for a sporty little Mini Clubman. Just as she was starting to think it had been stolen, she found it. She walked over, really relieved, and zapped the car so she could get in and drive off. Nothing happened. She zapped it again. And again. And again. Still nothing happened. Shit, thinks Mam. I'm here in Ponty and I can't get into my car. Just then a man walked past and, seeing her in difficulties, stopped to offer some helpful advice. "The battery must have gone," said Pontypridd's answer to Jeremy Clarkson. Now if that were me, I'd have thumped him but Mam is more ladylike. "What can I do?" she said. "Well, I've never seen it done, but you can recharge batteries using magnetic waves from your brain power," said the man, "If you hold the key fob to your head and hold the button down for a few seconds, you can charge it up with your brain waves, and that should be enough to let you open the door."

Mam tried it. Nothing. "Perhaps you didn't charge it for long enough," said Mam's knight of the road (or the car park). "Give it another go. It'll work in the end." And with that, he went on his way, leaving Mam standing there holding her car keys to her head with the button held tightly down, then pointing it at the car and zapping it. But it wasn't working, so Mam started to panic. She walked to the entrance of the car park, looking worried, when two more blokes came up and asked if she was OK. She explained that she wasn't, and why, and they said: "Would you like us to have a go at getting into your car for you?" Now what would you do if two men you don't know offer to gain access to your motor vehicle which is locked? Well you'd just give them the car keys and walk away, wouldn't you? Of course you wouldn't. But Mam did, handing over the keys and walking off to phone me. When she told me what she'd done I was incandescent! "You've given your car keys to two blokes you've never met in a car park who offered to break into your car for you? Are you mental or what? We're coming down now. Geraint, get the car!"

So off we drove to Pontypridd, having told Mam we'd come with her to get her keys back, or call the police if the men – and the car – had gone. We arrived at the car park to find Mam, and we went to the car. The men hadn't been able to get in, but they'd waited by the car for her to give back the keys. So now we're there and the question is: shall we call the AA, or break one of the windows and open the car that way? But as I was looking into the car, something struck me. "Mam, haven't you got a picture of Dad on the dashboard?" "You know I have," she said. "So where is it?" She looked, and it wasn't there. Then she looked at the car again. Someone must have taken her personalised number plate too, because that wasn't on the car. "You've been trying to break into the wrong bloody car," I said. Thank God she hadn't succeeded, because if she'd told this story to the police they'd have had her in front of a magistrate before you could say "Not guilty". Or, worse, they might have believed her and called for a doctor.

**The one with the poo on the wheel**
Jeremy could have been forgiven for thinking that some of the stories were made up because they were verging on the ridiculous, but this one he actually saw for himself. I had been telling him about one particular client who was coming in on that day, and how she always brought her children with her. And whenever they came, they turned the place upside down with colouring books, drinks, food, little computers and other toys. At that moment, the woman arrived with her two kids in tow. Well, one was in tow, the other

119

was being wheeled in in a very expensive push chair. Immediately the shop began to resemble war-torn Beirut as books, toys and clothes were strewn everywhere. Now the floor of the shop is always kept spotless – hence Avalon's mishap with the sweeping brush – and I was a little bit concerned when I saw a suspicious dollop of something of a strangely brown colour on one of the thick tyres of the pushchair. The last thing I wanted was to see a trail of shit wheeled through the shop – apart from anything else I had no idea what Avalon could do with a wet mop – so I put on my best customer service adviser voice and said: "Oooh, that looks like something nasty on the wheel. Were there dogs about outside? You must have gone through it when you were crossing the road. It might be a good idea to clean it off now; the last thing you want is to get that on the carpet in your boot, as it'll be a bugger to clean off and it'll smell."

I thought I'd been pretty clever, making it all about my concern for the poor woman's car mats, and I expected a quick clean up, but I wasn't prepared for what happened next. The woman immediately dropped to all fours, put her head right up close to the tyres and took a good, long sniff. "It's OK," she said. "It's only mud."

Now, with my senses in overdrive, I couldn't have done that. I'm just glad that she had a good sense of smell, because I was afraid she was going to lick it!

These are just a few of the tales that get bantered back and forth every day, with the girls taking it in turns to be the heroines of the stories, or the butts of the jokes. It's all good fun, and the customers love it. It's like being in a West End play, where every actor is word-perfect all the time – it's just too good to miss. And that's why I love going there: it's just like going home. Because it is my home.

# Chapter Twelve

### Friends and Family

Friends are relatives you make for yourself
***Eustache Deschamps***

For some time after I was diagnosed with cervical cancer, Geraint and I didn't tell anyone about it, except my very close family – Mam, Kath, Steve and Avalon – and only gave the most limited of information to the boys. In the case of the boys, I suppose I just didn't want to worry them, especially given that I was sure I was going to get better. In the case of my wider circle of friends, I didn't want to be the object of pity. I've said already that I didn't want to be the guest of honour at anyone's pity party, and no matter how hard people try, they always treat someone differently after the word "cancer" is mentioned. And I didn't want that to be me. So I told very few people.

I suppose I have never had a huge circle of friends – but then who does? I do have a few really good friends and then a much larger circle of acquaintances. Now some of these are really close to me, but others are less so, and strictly speaking they are not really friends at all. I imagine a few of those might be disappointed to discover that I see them more as acquaintances than friends, but that's often just the way it is. And I think that I was more open about my condition to friends than acquaintances, which sounds logical, but, not even all of my friends were brought into the loop early on. As time went on, the number of people I told about my diagnosis increased, but there were still some real friends who I didn't break the news to for a very long time, and I know that many of them wish that I had said something so they could have helped in some way. To them I can only say sorry. The last thing I wanted to do was hurt anyone's feelings, but once I was diagnosed I had to deal with the positive aspects of treatment, and getting well for my family and myself. That had to be my main priority and I didn't want, or need, to be sidetracked. I think – I hope – my friends can understand this. It really wasn't personal, and wasn't as if I didn't feel close enough to them to tell them. To use an old saying, the ones who matter won't mind, and the ones who mind don't matter.

Among the people I did tell were the girls in the shop, who knew fairly soon that something was wrong. Telling them was the right thing to do, because they are very close to us and also because they would understand if Mam or Avalon had wobbles. In any case Tarryn and Kate are family. I'm not going to name the other people who were burdened with my secret here, but suffice to say all were asked to keep it confidential and all did. They were able to give me support when I needed it, and didn't put me under pressure at any time, either about my plans to go off to America and the course of treatment I was following, or the decision not to go down the medical route sooner.

Over time, news of my cancer has got out – I haven't gone out of my way to conceal it – and people have all been wonderful. The gossips who spread those rumours about me getting a gastric band certainly made my day, and you have no idea just how funny I thought that was. But you can understand their point – formerly large woman has massive weight loss after

123

going to a Florida health retreat for three weeks. Liposuction and a rubber ring round the stomach would be quite high on the list of potential reasons, I suppose.

Living up near Brecon now, I tend to come in most mornings with Geraint and the boys for school and then go to the shop, so my immediate support network and the friends I spent most time with are the girls from Mam's shop. We're a happy bunch: the girls styling hair and talking to the customers, me sitting on the sofa with my feet up drinking coffee and all of us chatting and watching the world go by. But there are a number of others who I spend lots of time with.

A lot of my time is spent with the Cricket Wives, which may make us sound like the Real Housewives of Dowlais Top, but we're not really like that. We're just a group of girls whose husbands, sons or both play for the same club, and who socialise together at matches and outside that. It's the sort of thing that happened a lot in South Wales at rugby clubs over the years, where players' wives – and sometimes mothers – used to prepare meals for the teams, and it was really an extension of the socialising that happened anyway. That sort of things doesn't happen so much with small rugby clubs any more, but it is still a big part of cricket, where cricket teas are so well organised.

But if that makes it sound like we only spend time together because our sons and husbands do, well nothing could be further from the truth. The cricket matches may give us the means and the opportunity to get together, but we don't need a motive as we all get on really well. Besides which, I've known many of the girls for years outside cricket, too. For example, one of my closest friends, Claire Stanfield-Davies, is also the practice nurse at the Morlais Medical Practice, the doctors' surgery I attended in Merthyr. When I was first diagnosed and hadn't made any announcements, she kept my confidentiality just like the professional and the friend that she is. But once she had become involved in my care, she did tell me: "If you'd prefer someone else to look after you at the surgery, I really wouldn't be offended. I wouldn't want things to be awkward or embarrassing for you because we are close."

"Not a bit of it," I said. "If someone has to be seeing my bits, I'd sooner it was someone I know rather than a complete stranger." Claire and I have known each other for donkeys' years, ever since we were teenagers together, but we have really got close in the last five or six years as we both have boys who played in the same team at Hoover's Cricket Club, and her husband Wayne is a friend of Geraint's too. She was absolutely mortified when I told her that I was going to Hippocrates for treatment rather than adopting the conventional route, but she still didn't try to dissuade me from going. "Do that but have the radiotherapy treatment too," was how she put it. Later on, when my oncologist was talking about chemotherapy following the radiation treatment, Claire told me: "You'd better be having it." When I told her that I was, she was very pleased: "I hoped you'd be going for the stronger option (paclitaxel), but one type is better than none." It must have been hard for her, having to respect my confidentiality and not say anything in front of people who didn't know and who might have been speculating as to what was going on in my life. She is a woman of strong opinions – just like me, which is why I love her so much – and she has called me a silly cow on more than one occasion, but has always been 100% supportive of me,

Claire is my closest mate among the Cricket Wives, but the others are also regularly in touch: the two Janes

–Clement and Thomas – Julia Barry, the Sians – Morgan and Parfitt – and Judith Whatley. They ring regularly to see how I am and if there's anything I need. Through the summer we are together most weekends, though last season that happened quite a bit less after I was diagnosed. Outside the season, we've met a few times for lunch – like that time in Alfred's when I ordered the scallops!

During the last year I have also become very close to the girls from Cancer Aid Merthyr Tydfil, where I go for my aromatherapy treatments. Cancer Aid is a local charity, staffed by 60 volunteers from the borough and further afield who are doing their bit to make cancer sufferers' lives just that little bit more bearable. I go there for my aromatherapy, but in addition to that the charity offers a range of other services, including providing transport for cancer sufferers who have to attend hospital appointments for radiotherapy or chemotherapy treatments and don't drive, especially as Velindre and Llandough are not on the main railway lines or bus routes, and early appointments can't always be served by public transport anyway. A network of fundraisers generates cash to keep the centre and a shop, purpose-built and recently opened in Dowlais, operating. During the time I've been going there I've become close friends with Yvonne Jones; Tracey Burke, the centre manager; and Rhiannon Harris, who does my aromatherapy.

I've known Yvonne for years – her son plays rugby with our boys and she is a cancer survivor herself. Her brother coaches one of the age-grade teams up at Merthyr RFC as well, so he and Geraint know each other well. Tracey has worked for Cancer Aid for thirteen years, starting off as a volunteer and working up the ladder to become Centre Manager. She got involved after losing her father to cancer years ago, so she knows what it is like to watch someone you love fight an illness that may have many side-effects, both physical and psychological – and not just on the cancer sufferer.

Rhiannon and I connect on a spiritual level – she does holistic therapies up at the centre and is very knowledgeable about pressure points, as one would expect from a black belt martial arts fighter. She knows a lot about other holistic therapies and I'd like to think so do I, so we talk a lot about things. And we really connect: once she did Reiki on me and actually had to leave the room to sit down! Afterwards she told me that she had felt so much power coming through me that it almost knocked her sideways, and that if she hadn't left the room she knew that she was going to collapse. The next time she did Reiki on me, I think she was a bit more cautious and careful.

Rhiannon does reflexology too, and is very good at reading my feet. But every time she does me, she keeps telling me: "I can't find anything in the feet." Some of you may have heard about reflexology but not really know what it is all about. Basically, it is an alternative medicine involving the physical act of applying pressure to a patient's feet, hands or ears with different finger, thumb and hand techniques. It is based on what reflexologists describe as a series of zones and reflex areas that reflect an image of the body on the feet and hands, and they work on the premise that applying pressure to different areas brings a physical change to the body. And when Rhiannon applied force to the pressure points relating to the cervix, she was not getting any indication of a disability or any illness, which is why she could not feel my cancer. Now this may sound stupid, but I was told the very same thing by Judith Whatley, who is herself a Reiki practitioner. She's also done my feet and couldn't find anything present, and remarked herself that it was all very odd.

Of all the people who have helped me though this, the one I haven't mentioned here yet is my closest, my very best friend. Geraint has been my rock, the one constant at this time of craziness and uncertainty. It has been hard for him to see the pain in my eyes every day as he's watched me dealing with my cancer. He was with me when Dad went through it, and his dad, Eddie – another larger-than-life character – also lost his life to cancer so he's got some experience of what can happen, and in many ways that must make things worse for him. And he's had experience of dealing with cancer in a different way. Both his dad and mine were men of their time, I suppose you could call them old-fashioned if you like, but definitely different to me. Their way of dealing with cancer was by not talking about it, and trying to be strong for the people around them by not making it a part of their loved ones' lives. But every step of the way, I have talked through all our options with him, and he's been 100% beside and behind me in the treatment options I have elected to follow.

When I was diagnosed – in fact even before I was diagnosed – Geraint could tell there was something wrong with me, the way that old married couples can instinctively feel their partner's pain. He had encouraged and urged me to go to the doctors' for a long time before I did, but I'm stubborn and I tended not to listen. And as I've said before, the menopause was a handy – though, as it turned out, wrong – diagnosis on my part.

We have been married for 20 years, and together for longer than that. Geraint likes to tell the story of how he saw me in a pub in Merthyr one evening and told his mates: "That's the girl I'm going to marry", which took a lot of balls for a 16-year-old who may have been overindulging in the beer a little when he saw me, a few years before he was legally allowed to go into a pub and buy a pint. Not only was I three years older than him, but I was just about to go off to America to work, so his confidence might have seemed more like cockiness – but here we are, a quarter of a century down the road, still together. Now when you've been with someone for as long as we have, you can tell what they might be thinking, and I can say with my hand on my heart that since I was diagnosed – and before that even – there hasn't been one day when Geraint hasn't been up and ready to go with me to face whatever that day may bring. As he said: "There've been days when I haven't wanted to go to work, but that's only so I could be with Annmarie and help her with the boys." I know that the boys and I come first in his life, though sometimes he tells me cricket comes first, but I don't believe him.

At the time I started to feel ill, Geraint was running his own business fitting synthetic outdoor floor surfaces, but it soon became hard to support me and run his own show so he packed it in and started working for my property developer brother-in-law, Steve, as a site manager. As things got worse and I was diagnosed, though, he took a sabbatical to look after the boys and me while I get well. It hasn't been easy for me, and I have absolutely no idea how I would ever have coped without him. He's effectively turned into me, and has taken on all my duties. The downside of this, of course, has been that because Geraint has been looking after the house, he has not been earning any money. We ate into all our savings pretty spectacularly, and luckily we have had lots of support from the family – they have been magnificent.

My illness has transformed Geraint about the house too. I've already about written how he looks after the

129

boys, a responsibility he took on when I went to Hippocrates and has continued to shoulder ever since. He was never a lazy man; he's worked hard ever since I've known him, but he wasn't a natural in the kitchen. I think it's a product of the time we grew up in where the men worked and the women ran the house. Kettles, toasters, ovens, washing machines: they were things he walked past in Curry's, or helped plumb in whenever we got a new one, but the actual operating of them tended to be my responsibility. But that changed swiftly and to be fair, he's not looked back. Nothing holds any fears for him now, and he cooks meals from scratch. Not bad for a boy from the Valleys in his 40s ...

# Chapter Thirteen

## The Secret

*No pessimist ever discovered the secret of the stars or sailed to an uncharted land or opened a new heaven to the human spirit*

***Helen Keller***

I was watching daytime TV one day, soon after I'd come back from Hippocrates, the way you do when you're killing time waiting for another programme to start, or for someone to call in to see you, and was idly flicking channels and I came across a repeat of *The Oprah Winfrey Show* from 2006 on Sky (I can't remember which channel). As she is my heroine, I stuck with her. She often has interesting guests, I thought, so why not?

As I started to listen, I realised she was talking about a self-help book that has subsequently gone down a storm in America – because it was featured on two episodes of Oprah's show – called *The Secret*. And it must have been good, because Oprah, who is no stranger to dramas and upheavals in her personal life, said: "This book changed my life." As I listened to the programme and the people talking about it, I came to wonder if it might change mine too. We are all looking for signs, and as you know I tend to see symbolism in dates – and Oprah said that the book changed her life on May 24. That's my birthday! Surely that had to mean something.

*The Secret* is a best-selling 2006 book written by Rhonda Byrne. It is based on the law of attraction – the idea that "like attracts like" – and argues that life-changing results such as increased wealth, health and happiness can be brought about by positive thinking. Byrne wrote that as we think and feel certain emotions, a corresponding frequency is transmitted into the universe, and this brings back events and happenings and circumstances to us that are "on" that same frequency. As a simple example, if I think angry thoughts and feel angry, then Byrne would say that I attract back events and circumstances that will make me feel more anger. The opposite is also true though, Byrne believes: so if I think and feel positively, I will attract back positive events and circumstances.

It sounded interesting, certainly interesting enough for me to want to know more, so I went to the computer, clicked on to Amazon.co.uk and ordered a copy, which arrived the next day. I read it all in one sitting – I only stopped to make myself something for lunch; I literally could not put it down and was hooked. Since then, I've bought and passed on more than 20 copies of the book to friends and family. I bought a second copy for Geraint, and ones for Mam, Kath and Avalon, and many other people. I gave a copy to anyone that I thought needed to glimpse some light at the end of the tunnel. In fact, I bought so many that Amazon banned me from buying the book – they must have thought I was operating as a bookseller, getting copies cheaply off them and reselling to make a profit!

I really think that it is a powerful book, and it has had a huge impact on the way I live my life, and the way that I have dealt with my cancer. I've always been able to see future events – I think I was a little bit psychic even before I knew what being psychic meant

– and I've always tried to be positive about it. I always knew that I was going to get cancer, just as I know now that I will beat it – and I have always been positive about that, but *The Secret* just reinforces my belief that this is the way to deal with cancer – or with any type of problem: if you are positive, things will work positively for you. And in my life, the proof is out there. I have my vision board, and I'm always removing things from it as I achieve them, and I have my barn, which was something I always wanted, and even as events seemed to conspire to prevent it from coming true – first the owner of the original barn's refusal to let us film our audition tape there, then the shelving of the programme followed by my illness and finally the cancellation of the show –we came through in the end, even if it was with a different barn.

I summed this up in a short piece I wrote as a guide for myself:

*I wish for health, peace and harmony and contentment for all my family.*

*I wish for prosperity, for happiness and love and to pass the gift of the secret on to as many others in the knowledge that it will make a difference to some lives but also understand that it can't reach all – it is not for everyone.*

*I am thankful for my belief and look forward to each new day and the experiences that I receive.*

This is how I have faced my cancer, by being positive and knowing that I will come out on the other side. And while Geraint, Mam, Avalon and all the others may not have been able to get as much from *The Secret* as I have, where it has helped them is that they can see where I am coming from and what my approach to my life with cancer is.

When I was diagnosed, I started off with a holistic approach, looking to heal my body and spirit together, and this took me to Florida and the Hippocrates Institute. I am convinced that the only reason this did not work for me is that I wasn't able to follow the dietary approach through to the full because my body wasn't able to handle the tastes and smells of the fresh vegetarian products. The failure was mine, not Hippocrates'. When it became apparent that this first step had not worked, I went for radiotherapy as I felt this would give me the best option of curing my tumour without massive side-effects, but when that ultimately failed to halt my cancer's growth then I underwent chemotherapy. And though it all, I remain convinced that I will be cured. No doubts or "what if's" for me.

But while I am the most positive person I know, I am also something of a realist, so "what if" also had to be considered if only to ensure that we had the contingency covered. Now before I began having chemotherapy, my oncologist, Louise Hanna, outlined the procedure as we talked about how many treatments I would or should have. Having seen how the paclitaxel sapped my dad's strength, I definitely didn't want that to happen to me, so we agreed that we would review the treatment after three cycles of chemo. Normally at this time, after three or four treatments of chemotherapy, you will have an MRI scan to determine what effect the treatment has had on the tumour. This then gives the doctors the opportunity to decide on what to do next. "What to do next" can mean a number of things, such as continuing with another few cycles of chemotherapy because it has shrunk the tumour or make changes to the chemotherapy drugs because it has not worked as well as hoped for. There is one other "what to do next", of course – and that is to discontinue treatment.

Right from the beginning, I had said that I never wanted to let the treatment for my cancer affect my quality of life any more than it had absolutely had to, and to a large extent this view was shaped by Dad's cancer. So we agreed right from the get-go that we wouldn't flog a dead horse. If after a course of chemotherapy, the tumour had not shrunk then it was pretty certain that the treatment had failed and we would not continue beyond that point. So after the third cycle of treatment in August, there was a wait while an MRI scan revealed how my treatment had gone. If the cancer had shrunk, then we continued; if not, then …

As you can imagine, there was quite a lot riding on the outcome of the review meeting, scheduled for September 17. "What if…?" had to have been in the back of my friends' and family's minds, no matter how confident we may have been, and the trip to get my results after the scan was quite a nervous one. Whatever I was going to be told would change everything, one way or another, in a pretty major way. Had the tumour shrunk? Or had it got bigger? Or even, as a fluke, had it stayed the same size? But the unpredictability of life continued to throw us curve balls. As far as I was concerned, the result that we got was one that I'd never considered getting – the scan was inconclusive. Geraint maintains that it was the chip I'd stolen from his portion of fish and chips from the Top Gun Fish Bar in Whitchurch an hour or so before I had my scan that skewed the reading – I'm sorry, but it smelled (and tasted) delicious! Whether or not that's true, I'm not sure, but whatever it was it certainly messed up our thinking – not to mention the scan!

What was I to do now? Things hadn't got worse,

which was a plus. But they hadn't got better either, had they? On the other hand, they might have done either – or they might have stayed exactly the same. The worst thing about this result was that we just didn't know what it meant, and that was a problem because the outcome of this scan was supposed to determine what I was going to do next. We had already agreed the strategy that we would follow: if the tumour had got bigger I was going to halt chemotherapy rather than subject myself to a course of treatment that would gradually increase its effects on my body, making me more tired and suffer from diarrhoea and stomach upsets for longer and longer each month. True, thus far the effects had been negligible – but I knew that the greater the number of chemos I endured, the more these side-effects would probably increase in both the length of time they affected me and their severity. And I didn't want to go down the route of seeing my life as a succession of weeks in bed with occasional good days, as opposed to what I had now which was the very opposite.

However, we had also agreed that if the tumour had not grown in size then the treatment was, at the very least, stopping it from spreading further; and if that was the result of the scan then I would continue to undergo chemo for a further series of treatments and see what the next scan showed. And the result we had got now – which was effectively no result – was more like the tumour not having grown than any other. If it had got bigger or smaller, then the scan should have been able to detect that and it couldn't. So, in the absence of any more concrete guidance, I went on with my treatment, hoping that the next scan would show more positive results.

And so it was that in November, I completed the first course of chemotherapy (I've had a total of six to date), and had a blood transfusion to help boost my red blood cells because I was anaemic. It sounds scary, to think that I needed blood – but it wasn't really. Anaemia, which is a reduction in the number of red blood cells in the body, affects many people with cancer at some time during their illness. Some people get it because of the cancer, but I got it as a result of the chemotherapy (it can also be caused by radiotherapy too). Anaemia can lead to tiredness, a loss of energy and, in some cases, breathlessness; this happens because red blood cells contain haemoglobin which carries oxygen around the body. People who are undergoing cancer treatment have their haemoglobin level tested, and if it is low, as it was in my case, a blood transfusion may be carried out. Other than that, the side-effects thus far had not been awful, I would say, but they were getting stronger and longer-lasting with every cycle of chemo, so that was something to take into account when I next talked to Louise Hanna.

My next scan was scheduled for the beginning of December, with a meeting to discuss the results on December 13, two weeks before Christmas. So there I was on my way back to Velindre to see Louise once more, travelling in a caravan of Christmas shoppers heading towards Cardiff. But while their big decisions centred on the latest gift ("Which tablet shall we buy? iPad or Nexus?") potentially my decisions would be far more influential.

Geraint and I had been positive throughout – but given the pain I'd been having as the tumour pressed on my sciatic nerve and the additional problems it was causing me with drop foot syndrome, which made walking without a stick well-nigh impossible, the prospect of bad news was in the back of our minds.

And so it proved. Louise was straight, as was her way – something we have always appreciated. The tumour was growing, despite the additional course of chemo I had undertaken when the previous scan was inconclusive. She didn't say how much it had grown, and I didn't ask: all that was important for us to know was that it was increasing in size.

So three months on, I was faced with the same question that had confronted me after that inconclusive scan: what do I do now? Louise outlined my options, of which there were really three: chemotherapy, but this time with paclitaxel (the taxol-containing drug), the very thing I had been determined to avoid; chemotherapy with another drug which, while stronger than carboplatin, is not quite as toxic as paclitaxel; or discontinue chemotherapy altogether. And it really was something of a lottery, because Louise told me, after she'd outlined the options available to me, that she didn't really know just how beneficial they would be, if at all.

So what was I to do? As Geraint and I drove back from Velindre, we kicked the possibilities around in the car. Well paclitaxel was an option, but how much of one was it really? A course of paclitaxel wasn't a good thing to undertake as one of its side-effects is that it affects nerve endings, and as I already had drop foot affecting my left leg I couldn't risk losing the use of my right leg too: I wouldn't be able to walk as I wouldn't be able to feel my feet. Add to that the tiredness and hair loss and I'd be suffering the very thing I had been so determined not to go through. As for the slightly less toxic drug, even if that did not have quite so many – or quite such severe – side-effects, there would still be some. And when all was said and done, it might all be for nothing.

As for giving up on treatment ... back in 2012 when I first decided to try chemotherapy, it was after Louise Hanna told me that my condition was very, very serious. She didn't give me a timescale, but from what she had told me I went back and did some research with my friends Yahoo! and Google and worked out that by her reckoning I had about four months to live – and even then she said that the treatment might have no influence on the final outcome. Well, I thought as we drove home, I've already had two more months than that. If she had been right I wouldn't have seen December and yet here I am almost at the beginning of a new year, alive and kicking – even if it's only on one leg.

I'd backed my judgment so far, with Geraint's advice and support, and between us I think I can say that we had defied medical predictions. But this next decision was important, so I decided … not to decide. Rather than make a snap decision in December, we decided that I'd give myself a break from the chemo to let my body recover, and then make a decision in the New Year about what to do: whether to undergo another course of chemotherapy or to stop having treatment altogether.

When we came home, we told Zack that we were taking a break before deciding what to do next, and he was fine about it. We didn't say anything to Harrison, Harvey and Roddy other than telling them that I was having a treatment break to recharge my batteries. After all, there wasn't anything to tell them right now – and in any case, that was exactly what was happening.

We told Mam, of course, and the girls at the shop, and they were fine about it. Mam though, was a starting to be a little bit in denial. If anyone asked her about how my cancer treatment was going she would say: "It's not cancer, it's sciatica!" I think that, in her mind, she was not associating the thing that was pressing against my sciatic nerve with the tumour I had been receiving treatment for.

Some people may think that by taking time out before making a decision about future treatment, I was acting like a rabbit caught in the headlights, paralysed and unable to move. And while that might be true of some people, that just wasn't the case with me. Taking a breather before deciding seemed like exactly the right thing to do, for so many reasons. To start with, there was my general health to consider: in myself I felt fine. People who don't know me and who came into the shop had no idea that I'd been ill – obviously people who knew me when I was much heavier will have seen a change in me, but to the world at large I didn't look like someone at death's door. Even my oncologist, Louise, who knew my condition inside out, said to me: "I have to say it, you look a very picture of rude health." So, if I could fool her, I could fool anyone! Apart from feeling tired, which is a side-effect of the chemo, and the stomach upsets (which I still get from time to time), I was pretty chipper. As for my morale, well: while there have occasionally been 'down days', they are more like down hours, and I soon bounce back. Well, you've got to, haven't you? It's the positive thinking coming into play – it's *The Secret*.

And that's the thing. We have been positive throughout, Geraint and me. There's no denying that facing this has been hard, and sometimes frightening. Being diagnosed with cancer isn't something that you can just shrug off – but as I said many pages ago, it doesn't have to define you either. And whenever one of us has had a wobble, the other has been able to keep us on course. Together we've done the same for our friends and family and in return they have done the same for us

And being positive meant that when we finally decided what option to take – whether to go ahead with further treatment or say "enough's enough" – we'd be able to make the decision knowing that whatever we chose would be the right thing to do, even if it meant saying that I wouldn't undergo any further chemotherapy. But making that decision was some way in the future.

Making that call would be daunting for some, and even scary. But I wasn't daunted or scared. I was thinking positive thoughts and concentrating on bringing positive emotions, events and happenings back to me and mine. If I do that, everything is going to be all right – that's my secret.

## Chapter Fourteen

### Another Christmas in the Trenches

God, grant me the serenity to accept the things I cannot change, the courage to change the things I can, and the wisdom to know the difference

*__Reinhold Niebuhr__*

Christmas was coming, and while everyone else was shopping, I was trekking back down to the Royal Glamorgan Hospital in Llantrisant for another procedure – this time to have my stent changed. After all, I'd promised my surgeon, David Jones, my old one, rinsed out and gift-wrapped – too – and I am always a woman of my word.

Another reason why Christmas was different this year was that for the first time, the butler was being let loose in the kitchen. Before the event, Mam had suggested that everyone come to her because, as she gently told Geraint, cooking Christmas dinner was hard enough for a woman. But Geraint wasn't having any of it and, having done a "dry run" a week earlier, he was well up for the challenge. And the smell and taste were brilliant! I didn't eat as much as in years gone by, true, but the boys did. It must have been good too because Zack ate two dinners, even though the second was a bit of a struggle for him to finish.

By and large, though, Christmas was quiet, which is how we like it anyway. On the Friday after Christmas,

Jeremy and Annette came up to visit and I received them like the lady of leisure I was, in my *boudoir*, with my faithful retainer Geraint rushing up and down two flights of stairs bringing me coffees, toasted sandwiches and refills. A good time was had by all! New Year's Eve was something different again, as it was much more of a family affair when Kath and Steve arrived with the twins to see in the New Year. I was in bed with the girls clambering all over the place, and Steve brought a karaoke machine, flashing lights and all, into the bedroom. And to borrow a phrase from Geraint, "excellent was not the word".

After all that excitement I was hoping for a quiet start to 2013 but as the New Year progressed I started to feel a little under the weather and began to have difficulty passing water – in fact I hadn't peed since the Thursday evening – and on the Saturday afternoon, Geraint insisted that I go back to Prince Charles Hospital. He was firm about it, but didn't make too much of a song and dance, which was just as well really, because he told me afterwards that he thought my kidneys were failing. We were in the new Accident and Emergency unit when Jeremy texted to see how things were and Geraint told him we were back at Prince Charles. By now I was on a drip, and while at this stage Geraint hadn't told Mam or Kath I was back in, the doctors hadn't worked out precisely what was wrong with me so there wasn't too much information he could give them anyway and they and we sat back to await developments. That night, we had booked to go out for dinner at the Felinfach Griffin Inn, with Ger's cousin Delme, Delme's wife Sharon, and Ger's old schoolmates Chris Jones and Rob Jones, and their wives Sue and Emma. Delme and Sharon had been up to Rhiwlas before, but it would have been Chris, Sue, Rob and Emma's first times. But instead of seeing our friends I was in hospital in the Gurnos!

By 8.30 that evening I was feeling really tired, but I had had an X-ray and was waiting for a CT scan to confirm what was happening, and Geraint told friends who rang and texted to check up on me that I was going to spend the night at Prince Charles. But within an hour, that decision had been shelved and I was being shipped off to Ward 8 of the Royal Glamorgan Hospital, though by the time I arrived this had been changed to Ward 3. Some people wanted to visit but while I was happy for them to come, this was soon cancelled, as I was told that David Jones would be coming in specially to see me. It seems that the doctors thought that the newly fitted stent was causing the problems, and that it might have become blocked.

The drama wasn't over for the night, though, because when he was driving back to Brecon to get some sleep (and the stuff I would need for my hospital stay), Geraint had a tyre blowout about 12 miles outside of Cardiff at 2am. Because the car only had a tyre-inflating kit and no spare wheel, he couldn't fix it himself and had to be rescued by the RAC – Ger isn't a member of "the fourth emergency service" – and sustained by a tasty packed lunch (or rather a packed midnight snack!) which was hand-delivered by Richard Galliers, a friend from Merthyr RFC, who had read Ger's distress call on Facebook.

I was oblivious to all this as Geraint turned up at hospital early on the Sunday morning in time for my operation. I will admit to having been a little impatient at first because I had hoped the op would have taken place first thing, but it wasn't until 1.30pm before they started taking me down to the theatre – I joked with David Jones that he had had waited to complete his round of golf or his lunch before coming in. But once I was in theatre, the procedure to replace the stent went fine. If only the same could have been said for my bed rest on the ward…

Jeremy called in to see me on Tuesday and he later described it as "challenging". I was one among many patients with a wide range of ages and different conditions. All through the visiting hour, Geraint and Jeremy were being asked by the elderly woman in the bed opposite me what the time was, when she was being taken home and whether she would be having something to eat before discharge – I think she mistook them for hospital porters (which looking at the size of them was not such a silly mistake to make!) Given the fact that I'd just undergone surgery, wasn't eating well and was waiting for my bowels to move, I thought I was fine, but Jeremy said that in the short space of time he was there, he could see that I wanted to get out and back home as soon as possible.

In the event, I wasn't allowed home until Thursday. They wouldn't let me out for a few days because my bowels hadn't moved since the operation (this often happens after surgery), and then they had difficulty taking blood samples to check that my kidneys were functioning OK, because the veins in my arm had contracted; I've always had crap veins and would be hopeless as a junkie! But once the staff did take some blood, they confirmed that the kidney function and ECG tests were both fine, so home I came.

Geraint drove me back home to Brecon, and the next few days were quite busy as he juggled looking after both me and the boys before I went back to hospital – this time Velindre – on January 16. I had an appointment with a physiotherapist to see if anything could be done about the restricted movement and pain in my left leg. And while the physio tried everything, it didn't seem to make any difference and my movement remained restricted. The following week however, my leg didn't handicap me as much because everyone's movement was curtailed, this time by a heavy blanket of snow across South Wales which made the A470 Brecon–Cardiff road difficult to navigate, if not downright dangerous to attempt. But attempt it we did, because I was scheduled to return to Velindre once more on January 25, this time for my "chat" with Louise Hanna

This chat was to make the decision, postponed since the middle of December, about whether I was going to undertake another course of chemotherapy. I don't think Louise was too surprised to hear that, following six weeks of thinking about it and talking things through with Geraint, I had decided against undergoing another course, but she suggested that we review things again in eight weeks. I don't think that my closest friends were surprised that I had passed on another course of treatment because they knew how things were: in the particular place I had found myself in, any potential benefits could be achieved only by my undergoing the most aggressive regimen, with its associated extreme side-effects of tiredness, hair loss and the potential loss of sensation in my feet. I had always been against going down that route until that point, and even if I were tempted to give it a go now, Louise Hanna's words were in the back of my mind – that there was no guarantee that having the chemo would achieve anything. And that's not the most ringing endorsement when you are being asked to consider undergoing a very harsh treatment that is almost as devastating as the thing it's trying to prevent. I imagine that quite a few people can see my point there.

But while my decision not to receive more treatment meant that I was no longer suffering the draining effects of chemotherapy, my cancer continued to limit my mobility and sap my energy. Over a period of a few months, it had become progressively more difficult for me to get about, and in the New Year the trips to Merthyr for Mam's humour penicillin became more and more sporadic before tailing off altogether. However, not only was my mobility about town limited, it was also getting harder to move about the barn too – and it was really that lack of mobility that used to give me my "down days". Now Rhiwlas is really beautiful, and set into a hillside – which means that it has an internal slope and split levels on the ground floor (perhaps when it was a barn it had a root store or something beneath the main floor area). And what this meant was that once I came downstairs for the day, just moving from sitting room to kitchen and toilet would involve going up and down a flight of stairs. That would be child's play for me back in my prime, but now I was feeling weak with one numb foot, it was far too difficult to attempt on my own. And this – as in so many other cases – was where Geraint came in, where having him at home and looking after me was so invaluable. He spent so much time helping me up and down stairs, and I certainly couldn't have managed without him. We had already bought a wheelchair for me to be able to go out, and we had also got two Zimmer frames – one for the bedroom and one for the shop. However, stairs were my real nightmare.

While Ger could help with the up-and-down assistance, he could do nothing about the tiredness that made every day more and more of an effort. Slowly but surely, I found myself spending more and more time in bed and the bedroom, not least because it had all the things that I might need most: namely an *en suite* bathroom and television (after Christmas, we added a commode to the arrangement when getting to the toilet became more difficult). The bathroom was particularly well-equipped but once it became more difficult to get in and out of the shower, as well as standing for long periods of time, we fitted a bath lift – a marvellous invention. Geraint contacted Macmillan in South Powys, and along came Sally Hilton, one of two nurses who cover an enormous geographical area. It was Sally who organised the bath lift, and she also talked about the possibility of getting a stair-lift for Rhiwlas, so that I could at least come down to the sitting room.

We knew that local authorities would carry out modifications for people with disabilities and serious medical conditions, so early in February we applied to Powys County Council for grant aid to carry out a modification for the barn. What we were hoping for was a stair-lift to connect our bedroom with the ground floor, but despite it only being one floor up, the modification would require two stair-lifts as there was a landing between the two flights of stairs with several openings off – so one continuous lift could not be fitted. This, we thought, might be the stumbling block. And lo and behold, our application was rejected, though not on grounds of potential cost. No, it was my prognosis which meant that, as far as the council was concerned, fitting a stair-lift was not viable. But the Thomases are nothing if not determined (and if anything, the Jameses are even more bloody-mindedly so!) and neither Geraint nor I were prepared to accept defeat.

So once more unto the Internet, dear friends; and with a bit of searching plus some ringing around we identified a firm that was locally based – in Hereford – which would rent us the lifts we needed. We put down the deposit and paid the first month's rental, and a team of fitters turned up on March 6: we were now the proud owners of our very own stair-lift. And although

Powys council hadn't been able to help us, Macmillan gave us a grant of £350 to go towards the fitting and costs, thanks to Sally Hilton.

So there I was: mobile again, or at least far more able to get up and down the stairs. However, before I had a chance to take the electric wonder on a test drive, fate stepped in once more.

# Chapter Fifteen

## Thursday

The most important thing when ill, is to never
lose heart

*Vladimir Ilyich Lenin*

Pain was something I was dealing with on a daily
basis, with the sciatic nerve and numbness in my foot
being really bad. You will recall how I'd started off
using hot water bottles and then paracetamol and
ibuprofen. Over a period of time since then, my dosage
of painkillers had increased from the over-the-counter
medicines to much stronger stuff. I had been
prescribed the morphine drink Oramorph quite early on
but I refused to take it. However as the pain got worse
I tried morphine patches in the summer of 2011, and
finally MST (morphine sulphate) tablets and
Oramorph. Initially I was taking 30mg of MST twice a
day, but over time the dose rose steadily: 60mg, 90mg
and finally 120mg. Bad as it was, I was still handling
it, just.

But it was getting progressively harder, and one day
towards the end of February, I was sitting on the
commode when I just broke down in tears. Geraint
came in to see what was wrong and I told him that I
wasn't going to get through this – I said that I thought I
was going to die. But I didn't want to die at home; it
would not be fair on Geraint of the kids letting them

see me go downhill like that. I'd rather go into a hospice or something. A few days later, Tracey Burke and Yvonne Jones from Cancer Aid Merthyr Tydfil called up to see us at the barn – it was the first time they'd been up – and while Yvonne and I were talking, Geraint had the chance to talk to Tracey about what I'd told him; he had to talk to someone. Tracey said that she would look at options for getting me into some facility or other, possibly the new Mountain Ash hospital. Geraint also spoke to Sally Hilton about the possibility of my going into the Usk House hospice in Brecon.

Tracey and Yvonne's visit was memorable for another reason. Mam, ever house-proud, came up early on the morning that they were coming to give the barn a once-over to ensure all my surfaces were clean (I swear she uses a white glove to check for dust). She went into the downstairs bathroom and yeugh! – somehow there had been a blockage and sewage was flowing up into the shower from the drains. She and Geraint mopped up the mess, but then Mam decided that "clean" was not good enough – we had to clear the blockage once and for all. Apparently, she said, an old plumber's trick was to cover the plughole with a plunger and pump the toilet with a loo brush with a towel wrapped around it to make a really tight seal. Well Mam wouldn't get into the shower, so Geraint went in and held the plunger down and Mam started to push as hard and fast as she could. Well she certainly had the right idea – nothing came up the plughole. Unfortunately, I don't think she was expecting the jet of poo that shot up around the brush and towel and covered her from top to toe. Mam was not amused – I had a snigger though!

Now birthdays are very important events in my family, and they also tend to mark other happenings in a spooky way. In 2012, Roddy's 12th birthday fell on the day we moved from Merthyr into the barn in Brecon, but this year I was determined to spend the day at home with the family to mark his becoming a teenager. Unfortunately I hadn't reckoned on my condition stepping in to take a hand.

A week before his birthday, I had a fairly severe haemorrhage from my vagina, certainly serious enough for Geraint to call the doctor. As we were now living in Brecon, we had transferred our business from the Morlais practice in Merthyr to the more local Talgarth Medical Practice and a doctor came out from there. She treated me with tranexamic acid, a blood clotting agent which stopped the bleeding. However, while I was no longer bleeding, I did start to get confused and disoriented and was having difficulty with my co-ordination. Over the space of a few months, I had been collecting adhesive strips from pads by rolling them like a cigarette and putting an elastic band round them, then adding to the roll each day. Now however I found it difficult to manage the roll, even though it was quite big, and kept dropping it.

Then the day before Roddy's birthday I haemorrhaged again and another doctor came out. She said I needed to go in to hospital, but there was no way I was going to mess up Roddy's day. A district nurse came to take bloods and the following day the doctor rang again and asked where we wanted to go. I said "Velindre," and a little while after Roddy had done presents and cards, I took my first trip downstairs on the stair-lift and Geraint and I rushed as fast as we could to... Pauline's, so I could have my hair done. There was no way I was going to see the NHS with flat hair! The shop had just closed and Mam and the girls did my hair before I went down to Cardiff.

Jeremy and Annette were due to call in that

afternoon, and rang to check if we were there but they must have passed us while we were in Merthyr. The journey itself to Velindre was pretty uneventful, and I was admitted and taken on to a ward, but the staff decided to move me to a side room to give me more privacy and access to a lavatory. The staff took the usual bloods when I arrived and my haemoglobin count was 3.7 – the normal range for a woman is 12–15 and one nurse said that mine was the lowest she'd ever come across. But that's me, I like to set new standards!

Over the weekend they gave me six units of blood and my haemoglobin count rose to a more respectable level. Not only that but Geraint brought Zack, Harrison, Harvey and Roddy down to visit on the Sunday, and we had a family day together. Geraint's birthday was on March 12 and while we didn't get to celebrate as much as we'd have liked, we did as much as we could. The plan was for me to be sent home on the Thursday so I'd be home for Dad's birthday on March 15, but on Wednesday night I had another bleed and again it was quite a large one. Geraint had to break the news to Mam, as I was quite upset because I was looking forward to getting back, but you know me – I soon bounced back. More blood and tranexamic acid and I was right as rain.

The doctors and nurses on the ward were great, and it was really something of a Merthyr old girls' reunion because among my nurses were Julie Powell,her sister Sian John, Glenda James and Linda George. I knew Julie from pre-Velindre days too because she used to attend the same spiritualist church meetings as my nan. And I had my visitors to keep me company too – Geraint, Mam and Avalon, as well as Annette and Jeremy, Claire Stanfield-Davies and her husband Wayne, and others. When Annette and Jeremy called in on Friday evening, Geraint passed them in the corridor as he was putting stuff into the car before popping back to get the boys sorted, and he told them: "This is another chapter for the book!" Then they arrived at my room and saw Mam with her scissors, neatly trimming my bouquet of flowers before putting them in a vase! Jeremy looked like he'd walked into a madhouse or something. For Jeremy it was quite a reunion too, because Julie Powell had been in school with him back in the day, and normally the only place they saw each other was in Tesco. I'm so glad I was able to be of service!

Over the weekend the boys came down again and we had another day together, and everything went swimmingly. While the boys were there, there was a moment when they popped out from the room to get a drink leaving Geraint and me alone, and I got a bit tearful over Roddy – he's growing up so fast and is a teenager now, but still a little boy in so many ways. And as things had been good health-wise over the weekend, I was really looking forward to coming home – this time the prospective date I'd been given was Wednesday, March 20th.

But on the Monday morning I had another haemorrhage. I was given more blood and they gave me a CAT-scan to check whether or not there were any blood clots that would need to be attended to. I was clear, and the doctors offered to give me a blast of radiotherapy to try and stop the bleeding. I agreed and the following day had the treatment. Hopefully, I thought, that would do the trick.

And it certainly seemed to, I slept well on the Tuesday and I must have perked up sufficiently for Geraint to plan to go home to the boys and to sleep in Brecon on Wednesday, after spending the two previous nights in Velindre with me, before coming back on the

Thursday. Jeremy, Kath and Zack visited me in the afternoon, and the tiny room was packed because Geraint was there too, as well as a nurse giving me another unit of blood. Now Geraint, Zack and Jeremy would make one hell of a front row so you can imagine there wasn't room to swing a catheter in there. Not only that, but Kath and Zack were attacking catering quantities of food that had been brought in, while looking at invitation patterns on Kath's iPad Mini. They didn't need me to be there at all!

That night, I had another haemorrhage. I was given more blood and then some tranexamic acid. Thinks I to myself: "Here I am, a mother of four in my 40s from Merthyr, a good Catholic girl. I've just had my first tattoo and now I'm doing acid!" I think that I was pretty calm about things, but a lesser person might have been getting a bit pissed off by now. On Thursday morning, Geraint seemed to be getting a bit distracted – I think he was concerned that the radiotherapy which was supposed to stop the bleeding didn't seem to have worked – so I was pleased when Louise Hanna called to see us and talked us through the process, and said it might take up to a fortnight to kick in fully, and there was nothing stopping me having another blast in a few days. I was all up for that.

In the afternoon, Mam and Kath came to join Geraint and sit with me, and we just chatted for a while. Then Geraint decided, having been relieved by the James women and with some prompting from me, that as he'd not gone back to Brecon the previous night he was going to shoot off home for a couple of hours and get Harrison, Harvey and Roddy and have a night in with them. And just after 4pm, I shooed him out and off he drove, ahead of the office traffic to get up the valley.

# Chapter Sixteen

## Thursday (Part 2)

When you feel like giving up, remember why you held
on for so long in the first place

*Proverb*

Jeremy Flye writes: *Planning for every eventuality is
something that we all do; whether it's filling the
cupboard with some extra cans of beans and soup and
the freezer with a couple of loaves of bread in case of
snow, or collecting favours that you can one day cash
in, everyone has a contingency plan somewhere in
their life. But though I've always tried to follow this
motto, this was something I didn't do for this book. I
never thought I'd have to.*

*Yet here I am ...*

*This chapter was the one I never expected Geraint
would to have to tell, because I never thought that
Annmarie wouldn't be about to finish the book herself.
No matter how much I knew of her condition and no
matter how sick I saw that she was becoming from time
to time, I always felt she would be able to bounce back
– if not just as strong as before, then at least as strong
as she could be under the circumstances..*

*So why did I feel like that? Well, that was down to
Annmarie herself. That incredible sense of humour,
that indomitable spirit and the never-say-die attitude
never left her. Nothing had ever got the better of her*

*before, and she wasn't going to start now. Whether holding court in Pauline's hair salon, or propped up in my front room with a hot water bottle as we talked – well, she talked and I tried to keep up with the note-taking – or more recently chatting to friends in her bedroom as moving became more difficult and she spent more time at home in Brecon, she was the same old Annmarie, a real character. As sharp as a tack, funny as ever, warm, gossipy without ever being hurtful, caring and considerate of others. Had she been able to think herself better then you wouldn't be reading this now but rather something far more humorous and, well, fitting.*

*In the end though, strength of character and grit were not enough and as time went on and the cancer took hold, her body could not continue to honour the cheques that her mind was writing for her. But because of her strength of personality and her lust for life, even those family and friends who were closest to her – and they were hardly blind to her deteriorating health – surely still felt that if anyone was going to beat this then it would be Annmarie. Because even when she was tired or in pain, the light in her eyes, shining brightly, never went out.*

*Right now, just as I'm about to slip into another paragraph about how she was handling things, I can hear Annmarie shouting in my ear, telling me to stop pratting about and tell you what happened next. So let's get on and let Geraint take up the story ...*

The drive back from Cardiff was pretty straightforward and I was thinking about collecting the boys and what I was going to make them for tea when my phone rang. It was Kath, and what she said was like a shock to the system: "Ger, you'd better come back here now. Quick." A quick loop around the roundabout at the

Cyfarthfa Retail Park and I was heading south again, trying to get back to Velindre as fast as I could. Annmarie had had another haemorrhage and it did not look good.

When I arrived at the hospital they were trying to hook Annmarie up to drips and a blood bag but as this was going on, a consultant pulled me to one side. "I don't think we are going to stop this one," she said. I went out and told Kath and Pauline. They took it pretty much as you'd expect – they were hysterical to begin with but then pulled themselves together for Annmarie.

I knew that this day might come. It was only that morning that I'd messaged a friend who had texted to see how Annmarie was after her haemorrhage on Wednesday night: "If I'm being honest, I can't see her coming out of here unless they can stop the bleeding. I asked the duty doctor this morning how long it takes for the radiotherapy to work. She said 'normally 24 hours' – it's now 48!" After that though, I'd spoken to Louise Hanna and she had reassured us that it would take longer. But that was before this bleed, of course.

I phoned Zack to get him to come and join us, and then Avalon, and then we waited together.

The end, when it came just before 7pm on Thursday, March 21, was incredibly peaceful. Pauline and I were holding Annmarie's hands, me on her left and Pauline on her right. Her arms were stretched out to the ceiling, as if she was reaching out to something, but still holding us tightly. We said goodbye, and she pulled her mam and me to her to kiss us both. And then she fell asleep. As well as the family, there were doctors and nurses in the room with us and as we said goodbye, one of them had to leave the room in tears. Annmarie had obviously come to mean a lot to them all.

Poor Avalon and her husband John arrived just

moments later – they hadn't got to say goodbye but I know Annmarie was thinking of them and their children Amy and Jonathan too. I rang a few of our closest friends to tell them Annmarie had gone. All were devastated; I don't think they expected her to decline quite as quickly as she did, given how strong she had been up to that point. Then came the hardest part of the day – breaking the news to our three youngest sons.

Harrison, Harvey and Roddy came to the hospital about 8pm, and after I'd told them that their mam had gone, we all went in together to see her. Then I took the boys in one at a time, so each of them could say their own private goodbyes before going back to Pauline's.

I'm not going to share what they said in the still silence of that room: I know; they know; Annmarie knows; and God knows. I think that's enough for now.

# Chapter Seventeen

## Fields of Gold

Drink to me
*Pablo Picasso (last words)*

A fine Friday morning in April and we are sitting in church.

Just a stone's throw away from Pauline's shop on Brecon Road, St Mary's, Merthyr is full to the rafters. No mass was celebrated on this particular morning, but the church is busier than ever. People started filing in before 9am, an hour before the service was due to begin; within half an hour every pew is full and people are standing at the rear as well as packing the churchyard. Just as well it's a fine day for it; it won't rain. All dressed immaculately, the congregation could be here to celebrate a wedding. Only the presence of an oak casket resting in the transept gives the lie to that.

As the priest finishes speaking, the bearers – Zack, Harrison, Harvey, my brother-in-law Steve, my cousin Delme and Avalon's husband John – rise and take their places, three on each side of the coffin. Roddy, Pauline, Kath and I stand too to escort Annmarie on the final leg of her journey to the funeral cars that will carry her, and us, to lay her body to rest. I look at the mourners, and all I can see is a field of golden, yellow roses.

The coffin moves forward and Roddy, Pauline, Kath

and I follow, then the rest of the family as we leave the church, place the casket into the hearse and then take our seats in the funeral cars that will take us to Llwydcoed Crematorium, where Annmarie's father was cremated and where the final part of her funeral service will take place. And as we drive off, my mind goes over the events of the last few weeks. It's a fortnight since she left us, but time seems to have flown by …

Two weeks earlier, after we had all said goodbye to Annmarie in Velindre, the boys went back to Pauline's house with her while I stayed behind to complete as much of the paperwork and formalities as I could, before driving back to join them in Church Village. Everyone was heartbroken, but in some ways it was worse for Pauline because no one ever expects to have to bury their child; it's just not the natural way of things. So when I got to her house I was shocked by what I saw. There was Pauline, bustling about and getting on with preparing food for the boys. It was as if she'd decided for herself: "Right, Annmarie would not want me to sit about wallowing. My job is to look after my grandsons now." And look after them she did – she was amazing. I was expecting her to be numb - after all, we all were – and it was no time since she'd lost her husband to the same disease. But Pauline was like a rock.

The following day, I went back to Velindre with flowers and cards for the staff to thank them for the care and devotion they'd shown to Annmarie during her stay, as well as complete some of the paperwork it had not been possible to deal with the previous night. When I returned to Pauline's house, it was déjà vu as I walked in on Pauline, Father Michael St Clair, Avalon, Stuart Bush and his partner Janey McKenzie, and Gail Rees (another friend of Pauline's), who had called in

161

independently to pay their respects. Father Michael, who had conducted the funeral service for Roy, was also there to discuss preliminary arrangements for Annmarie. And just as happened when they were arranging Roy's funeral, everyone was … well, exceptionally well refreshed – let's put it like that.

On the Sunday after Annmarie died, Steve and Kath came up with Pauline to the barn and I cooked a family Sunday dinner. Our neighbours, farmers Anthony and Rachel, had given me a lovely rib of beef, which I cooked with locally produced vegetables. This was washed down with a bottle of the Louis Roederer Cristal champagne, which had become a family favourite, as we drank a toast to absent friends. After the last drop was drained, everyone wrote a message to Annmarie on small sheets of paper, and they were rolled up and put into the bottle and sealed: a fitting tribute to her, I think.

Zack was not with us. Before Annmarie had been taken in to Velindre he had arranged to go off to Belgium for a weekend with his mates, and I insisted that he went. He was a bit reluctant but it wasn't as if there was anything he could have done in terms of arrangements, and I know Annmarie would have wanted him to go. Amid the previous day's sadness, there was a moment of high farce because she had wanted to see him before he left with the boys – I think she realised it might have been the last time. So I left a message on Zack's phone but, rushing, I misspoke (as the lawyers say). "Zack, Mam wants to see you before she goes." I was mortified! I meant to say "before you go". Why can't you delete messages from a mobile phone before someone listens to them (or as Jeremy put it: "Why can't you find a *News of the World* reporter when you really need one?") Anyway, I was lucky. Like most men, Zack doesn't listen to his messages and saw that he'd missed my call, so rang me back and I was able to give him the correct message. After Annmarie died and we'd stopped crying and pulled ourselves together a bit, Zack listened to his messages on his iPhone. I guessed he'd got to mine when he said: "Bloody hell!"

I thought it was important to get the boys back into their old routines as soon as possible, and Zack's trip to Belgium was only part of it. So on Saturday, Harrison was back working in the music shop in Merthyr's Indoor Market, and in the evening he played a gig in The Crown pub with his band, The Canes. Harvey was being active too, having got into the Thomas family business: boxing. Back in February, he was robbed when he lost a points decision in a Welsh Championship boxing bout to a hometown jury at Swansea; but on Easter Sunday, he fought the champion again in a rematch, this time at Aberkenfig. The opponent may have been the same, but the fight definitely wasn't: Harvey remembered all the lessons from the previous fight, got stuck in early on and was a worthy winner. Roddy continued to put in loads of hours both with his golf and the Gwent cricket team, so there was a lot of driving to and from meetings and practice during the Easter holidays. On the Easter Monday, Kath, Steve and Pauline came up again, and we ate another family Sunday dinner, held 24 hours late because of the action-packed weekend.

After Annmarie died, people were incredibly kind and we had many cards, phone calls and messages from friends of ours, as well as friends of Annmarie's parents, Pauline and Roy, and friends of my parents, Eddie and Kay. During her illness, Annmarie had received countless letters and prayer cards from friends all over the world including one from a friend who had moved out to India; now many wrote a second time, but this time to offer their condolences. People called up to the barn to pay respects, and left many messages for me and the boys on Facebook. There were so many thoughts, expressions of sympathy and reminiscences that touched us that it would be wrong to single any particular one, but I have to mention one particularly heartfelt message which came from Julie Powell, who had nursed Annmarie at Velindre:

*It is always an honour to be with someone during their last days and hours. We had some laughs and, believe it or not, we cried together during those two days when nobody else was around. I had the privilege of being her nurse and friend and I will never forget her.*

The boys are rather quiet and reserved, so I hope he won't mind my repeating it, but Zack also put his fingers to the keyboard to let people know how he felt, and I feel what he wrote on his Facebook timeline is worthy of sharing here, as it is a great tribute to Annmarie and speaks well of her sons and the way she brought them up:

*Never really been too great at expressing thoughts/feelings openly, let alone writing them down. One thing I've always done was to say 'Thank you' and mean it to those that deserved it. As most of you know my mum lost her battle with cancer last week, despite her constant positive attitude and inner strength she'd fought for just too long. The last things she heard was me talking and the things I said couldn't have been more simple or more true – that I loved her and 'Thank you'. I wanted to thank her for everything from the qualities she'd given me to the things she taught me, the direction she'd pointed me towards in life and the amazing life she'd given me and my brothers in every way you could imagine. Thank you for being the best mum that anyone could wish for in my 22 years with her.*

*Also wanted to say a big thanks to the guys that I went away with on the weekend for keeping me sane and taking my mind off things.*

*Rest in peace Mam. Thank you for everything.*

Not a bad tribute, is it?

Funeral arrangements were in hand too. We had decided that Father Michael would take the funeral service, just as he had for Roy; the only difference now was that priests had been shuffled about and he was based in Chepstow. But that wasn't a problem, so he liaised with the family and Carwyn Iles, the 'son' from the funeral directors Raymond Iles and Sons, to complete all the arrangements. The working days that were lost over the Easter weekend threw the timescales for the arrangements a little, but we decided that the funeral service would take place at 10am on April 5 at St Mary's, and then over to Llwydcoed for the second half of the service and the cremation at 11am.

Annmarie had always insisted that she'd wanted to be "buried" as a Catholic, and while her attendance at church had fallen off in recent years, she was a believer. While she was in Velindre, the priest visited her on a number of occasions, and they prayed together. And on the day she died, after Louise Hanna had popped in to visit, the priest called again and Annmarie took communion with him, and asked him to give her the Sacrament of the Sick. I know that it would have been a great comfort to her then, as it is for us all now, that she was at peace with God when He finally took her.

Though almost all of Annmarie's funeral arrangements were very traditional, one particular instruction for mourners was inspired by her personal taste. In lieu of floral tributes and wreaths, the family had asked for donations to be made to Cancer Aid Merthyr Tydfil; they did so much for us and anything we can do in return would be scant payment for this (at the time of writing, donations in lieu of flowers have totalled £2,400). However, the funeral was not to be a flora-free affair: attendees were asked to wear a yellow rose – Annmarie's favourite colour for that flower – so that the proceedings would be no more sombre than they had to be. As we walked into church that day, the congregation had their backs to us so we could not see how many had complied. When we turned to face them and bear Annmarie's casket out, we were confronted by a host of golden blooms.

The morning of the funeral, we had decided to gather as a family at Pauline's house in Church Village and have the funeral cars collect us from there; it seemed the most sensible place to leave from as it was pretty much in the middle: between us in Brecon and Kath and Steve in Cowbridge. When we arrived, we were greeted with bacon and egg rolls for breakfast, and Kath had brought a couple of bottles of Cristal to wash them down with.

The week before, Kath and Pauline had taken the boys down to Cardiff to do any last-minute shopping and get bits and bobs – they took Zack's, Harvey's and my suits to the cleaner's, while Roddy and Harrison had new suits and all five of us had new pairs of shoes and white shirts – and when it was time to get dressed, it was like walking into the Wales dressing room at the Millennium Stadium: our clothes were laid out – jackets and trousers hanging up, shirts neatly pressed, shoes shined. And getting dressed for a funeral is a bit like putting on a suit of armour: it's like a ritual, and a bit of business that distracts and deflects you from why you are actually there. Then the cars came, and it was time to travel up to Merthyr.

Just before we went into church, my phone buzzed and a text came in from Claire and Wayne, who were unable to be with us for the funeral as they were out of the country, but who had to message to say that they were thinking of us. It was great to know that we were in their thoughts even though they were far away from Merthyr, so I replied at once before we went in. (I discovered later that one of Annmarie's friends, who had moved out to India, went to the Golden Temple in Amritsar to pray for her on the day of the funeral.)

In St Mary's, a close friend from cricket, Anthony O'Sullivan, read a passage from the Scriptures (1 Thessalonians 4, verses 13–18), which was incredibly appropriate:

*We want you to be quite certain, brothers, about those who have fallen asleep, to make sure that you do not grieve for them, as others do who have no hope. We believe that Jesus died and rose again, and that in the same way God will bring with Him those who have fallen asleep in Jesus. We can tell you this from the Lord's own teaching, that we who are still alive for the Lord's coming will not have any advantage over those who have fallen asleep. At the signal given by the voice of the Archangel and the trumpet of God, the Lord Himself will come down from heaven; those who have died in Christ will be the first to rise, and only after that shall we who remain alive be taken up in the clouds, together with them, to meet the Lord in the air. This is the way we shall be with the Lord for ever.*

*With such thoughts as these, then, you should encourage one another.*

We sang two funeral hymns at St Mary's – *Ave Maria*

and *How Great Though Art* – both of which were chosen because of their meaning to the family. *Ave Maria* was one of Annmarie's favourite hymns while *How Great Thou Art* was sung at Roy's funeral (you may remember the scene where Pauline drunkenly sang it to Father Michael because she couldn't remember the name of the hymn).

One change to the order of service worked in my favour. I had prepared an eulogy for Annmarie, and I was going to give it as soon as possible at the Crematorium as I wasn't sure if I would be allowed to deliver it in church, and I thought the longer the service went on the less likely I would be to do it justice as tears and emotion would take over. But Father Michael told me that I would be able to give it at St Mary's, so I was pretty relieved.

I'd written out what I wanted to say a few days earlier, but the only people I showed it to beforehand were my Uncle Cyril and Jeremy, and both said the same thing: "Don't change a word." So I didn't. I hope I made a good job delivering it as Annmarie deserved a fitting tribute. Anyway, here it is exactly as I spoke it:

*On May 24 1968, Roy and Pauline were blessed with the birth of their eldest daughter Annmarie, a beautiful, elegant, charismatic lady who would light up the room as soon as she entered. She had a very special bond with her family and would always be the salvation in times of crisis. Whatever the problem, she always found a way to resolve it.*

*I have known the family since childhood; my father cut the ribbon to open the salon and my mother was a frequent customer. Pauline and Roy came to London when my father had his MBE. So obviously I knew that along with Katherine, the Jameses had two beautiful daughters.*

I was 16 and standing at the bar of the Court of Requests and Annmarie walked in. I had built up a large quantity of Dutch courage through the evening so I approached her and asked her if she would like a drink which she accepted. Sadly she informed me that she was moving to America. I was devastated. I asked her for a goodbye kiss and she obliged.

I went back to my friends, and they were asking "who was that?" as she was 18 going on 19 at the time. I said: "Boys, that's the girl I'm going to marry". A difficult thing to do when she was living in North Carolina.

A few years later Pauline fell ill, and Annmarie came racing back from the States to look after her and the rest of the family. My parents had been invited to a ball in London by close friends of theirs; my dad was pretty ill at this time and had lost a bit of weight. He tried on his suit and it didn't fit him and he wouldn't wear a hired one in case the previous occupant had AIDS or something like that! So he wouldn't go. My mother asked Annmarie if she would go with me and she said yes. I felt like James Bond that evening, walking in to the Grosvenor Hotel with the most beautiful girl in the place.

The evening went well so I asked her for another date; she said yes and I took her to watch a Wales international football match (as you do!). That went very well, I thought – life couldn't get any better going out with a girl who is beautiful and loves sport! So I asked her to come and watch me play cricket for the day in Herefordshire, and again to my amazement she accepted. I had a pretty good game that day in Almeley, which I put down to Annmarie being there. She was definitely the one for me.

Some of the boys said this was a bad case of FGS – first girlfriend syndrome – but I knew she was the *special one.*

*I proposed to her and we had a magical wedding day. We have been blessed with four handsome sons: Zack, Harrison, Harvey and Roddy. Fortunately for them, they have inherited their mother's intelligence and good looks. Our boys have been our world; our life has been totally dedicated to them – and cricket! We have supported and chauffeured them all over the country for them to participate. Sundays mornings during the rugby season have been challenging when the four of them could be playing at different venues. Annmarie was a very vocal supporter and her shout of "Come on Merthyr!" will be ringing in my ears for many years to come.*

*Through the summer months cricket takes over, and it's not uncommon for us to be at a match of some kind every day of the week, and Annmarie would be there supporting us, in fact she has spent more time at cricket grounds than Geoff Boycott did at the crease!*

*A few years ago Annmarie's father Roy passed away. This was a difficult time for the family but again, in true Annmarie style, she picked up the pieces and made everything whole again, being the rock for her mother and sister and supporting our sons through that difficult time.*

*So when she was diagnosed, it was no surprise to me that she didn't want to tell anybody about her illness – especially the boys. She decided against having the conventional methods of cancer treatment as she saw her father suffer for 18 months with no quality of life. She wasn't doing that: she didn't want two years, five years, 10 years – she wanted to see her sons grow up and have grandchildren. She scoured the Internet and found a health centre in the States and decided to go there.*

*Things didn't work out like we had hoped and she*

turned to conventional treatment. While undergoing radiotherapy she volunteered us for making breakfast for the homeless at High Street Chapel: we would be up at 6am, do our chores then go to Velindre for treatment. She was amazing!

The past year has been a bit more challenging and she decided to move us to Brecon, hoping the fresh air and scenery would help her beat the illness.

The medical care Annmarie has been given has been first class. Louise Hanna and the nurses and doctors – especially the ones at Velindre – are worth their weight in gold and I can't thank them enough. Thanks, too, to Professor Jonathan Richards at the Morlais Medical Practice, the Talgarth Medical Practice, David Jones and the staff at the Royal Glamorgan, the chemo staff at Prince Charles and Nevill Hall hospitals, and Rob Howells and the staff at Llandough – we've done the full world tour in two years.

A very special "Thank you" to Tracey, Yvonne and Rhiannon and the rest of the staff at Cancer Aid. You have been a fantastic support to all of us; I'm so glad I found you. I can't thank our friends individually or we would be here all day. But thank you all for your continued support.

Annmarie never lost her spirit or dignity – the last time she left our house in urgent need of a blood transfusion at Velindre, she made me stop at the shop to have her hair done!

In her last moments, I held her left hand, Pauline her right with Kath and Zack there also. We said our farewells, and with her last bit of strength she pulled Pauline and me towards her and kissed us both. What a woman – a fantastic friend to Avalon, a caring granddaughter to Peggy, a loving daughter to Roy and Pauline, a wise counsellor to Kath and her family, a *magical mother to our boys and the most wonderful wife to me. You were simply the best.*

*Goodbye Princess. I promise to look after our boys and be the rock you were for the family.*

*God bless.*

After he'd read it, Jeremy told me it would take about six minutes to deliver; I don't know if anyone had a stopwatch on me but it felt like much less than that. I think it brought a few lumps to the throat – it certainly brought one to mine, and I knew what I was going to be saying. After that, the service continued to fly past as Father Michael talked at length about how Annmarie's life had been framed by three visits to St Mary's – the day she was christened, our wedding day when she made me the happiest man alive, and this final day when we had gathered to say goodbye. I think he struck just the right tone, neither too light nor too sombre.

I had been expecting a big turnout for the funeral, as Annmarie was very well known (as are both our families) but it was only when we took Annmarie to the car that I could see just how big. Before the service began, Carwyn Iles rang to say that the church was full by 9.30am and the turnout was greater than anticipated, so much so that they'd already run out of orders of service and had to print off another 150 copies.

The drive to Llwydcoed was short, far too short really, and when we arrived there seemed to be even more people lining the covered entrance to the chapel. We had decided that for Annmarie's last journey that the family would carry her in. Doing it was hard, but not doing it would have been even harder. We laid her casket on the plinth in the little alcove, and then took our seats for the committal.

At the front of the chapel was an artist's easel on which sat a beautiful portrait photograph of Annmarie taken by photographer Judith Cooke, one from a sitting that was to provide the jacket photograph for this book. It captured her spirit and sense of fun, and it was just like having her in the room with us. Which, of course, she was.

Before the committal, Steven Downes, one of our friends, led the mourners in singing *All I Ask of You* from *Phantom of the Opera*. This had been sung at our wedding, and Steven had sung it in the same place at Roy's funeral. Because it had so much meaning for the family it was only right to hear it again for Annmarie.

Then, after some more words from Father Michael and prayers, the service ended. But no closing of a curtain to signify the end of a life; instead, the strains of Whitney Houston's *I Will Always Love You* as people filed out. There were so many people that Whitney did more than five encores before the chapel was finally cleared! Then the receiving line ritual seemed to go on forever as so many people came to shake our hands and give Pauline and Kath a hug and a kiss. All had a warm memory or a kind word about Annmarie, and it's a tribute to her that so many came.

But it didn't end there. The traditional Valleys' funeral tea – or what one friend irreverently calls the AMF (after-match function) – was held back in Merthyr, in the Guest Keen Club in Dowlais, hosted by our friend Peggy Estabanez. The club is the old Guest Memorial Library, built by Lady Charlotte Guest to provide books for the workers of the Dowlais Ironworks and their families. Lady Charlotte is famous as the woman who translated *Y Mabinogion*, a collection of early Welsh myths and folk tales, from Welsh to English. There, beneath the easel and photograph of Annmarie, mourners mourned no more as they sipped pints and shorts, ate from the buffet and swapped tales and reminiscences. Annmarie would have loved it. (Although Lady Charlotte, and fashion designer Laura Ashley, are probably Merthyr's most famous and influential women, I bet she didn't have so many people turn up for their funerals!)

The beer and wine flowed, as did the stories, long into the night; and with the buffet long gone, we sent out for more food before a few hardy souls ventured into Merthyr itself. I was the last man standing, I'm pretty sure I was anyway. And I know my Princess would have approved; after all, what is more fitting than to celebrate a full life with a full day? Picasso knew what he was talking about ...

## Chapter Eighteen

### I Love You, Goodbye

**Meiji:** Tell me how he died
**Algren:** I will tell you how he lived
*The Last Samurai*

A friend of my parents, J Fyrsil Jones, gave them an anthology of his poems as a Christmas present back in 1994. One of them has always struck a chord for me:

*Think of me when I am dead*
*for my life shall be anew.*
*Wearied from this troubled world*
*– Joy will be my due.*
*These little words of comfort shall to*
*your hearts convey;*
*My fondest loving wishes*
*To you my friends – goodbye.*
*Prevent each precious little tear*
*With smiles and loving thoughts –*
*that we one day, will meet again,*
*in bliss beyond the way.*
*'Tis hard I know, yet do my will,*
*and let thy thoughts remember still*
*– those happy hours.*
*Remember me to love – kind and gentle.*
*I hasten, for my time is short.*
*Memories, sweet memories my friends*

*– Goodbye.*

It seems to capture, for me, the way we think about loved ones who have departed and how we need to focus on good memories that may often be distant days, rather than the often less pleasant, more recent ones.

In this spirit of reflection, I know that some people wonder how I feel now about Annmarie's decision not to undertake conventional medical treatment from the very beginning, rather than trying complementary medicine first, or not accepting the most aggressive treatments. Possibly they don't want to ask because they think emotions are too raw. But I'll happily tell you now, and it won't take long.

There was no way Annmarie would ever want her cancer to take over her life and that is what conventional medicine would have done. She had watched cancer take both her father and mine, and she was determined not to go the same way, where the treatment was not much better than the disease itself. She loved life and wanted to enjoy all of it for as long as she possibly could. I also genuinely believe that, had she been able to follow the healthy eating regimen laid down by Hippocrates, then it may well have worked; the failure was due to her inability to eat the food she was supposed to because of her 'dicky' tummy.

As far as I can see, the thing about cancer is that ultimately no one knows anything. Two people with the same cancer can be treated in the same way conventionally, so why might one person's treatment succeed and another person's fail? So even if Annmarie had gone for radiotherapy and chemotherapy straight away, would it have succeeded? Who knows? What we do know is that when she did finally go down that route, it did not work.

If I am bothered about anything, I'm far more bothered by the fact that Annmarie had never had a smear test. Not "hadn't had a smear test in the three years before her cancer was diagnosed", but "had never had a smear test". Now had her cancer been identified far sooner, it could well have been operable, and while we can never know what the outcome of that would have been, it is the case that surgery was never an option for her because by the time the cancer was diagnosed it was already at Stage IIb and inoperable.

So if you want to draw a lesson from my beautiful wife's death, then it is this: ladies, don't miss any opportunity to have a smear test. As soon as you get a reminder letter from Cervical Screening Wales or whoever provides your screening service, get onto your GP and book an appointment. Don't find out what is happening the hard way.

So that's it in a nutshell, the last few months of the life of Annmarie James-Thomas. I haven't gone into a great deal of detail about her last days for a couple of reasons. First, we all know someone who has succumbed to cancer, so we have a pretty good idea of how things go without hearing another story. Second, and more importantly in my mind, it really isn't anyone's business but her family's. Third, and most importantly: it's not what this book is about.

When Annmarie and I started this some months ago, she was very clear that this was to be an always positive, sometimes funny story about how she was making choices and squeezing the very last drop of life out of each and every day, not a chronicle of her illness (although, in charting the choices she made and the places she went, there has been some element of recording the progression of her cancer).

And even though she's no longer here, I want to follow the same path. I have no desire to tell you how

Annmarie died, but I hope this book will give you a small idea about how she lived, and who she was. I say "small" because there is no one quite like Annmarie. We're all unique, though many of us share character traits and behaviour, often with our closest family and friends. But I can say with hand on heart that Annmarie really was a one-off, a true original. And even though she came from Merthyr, a place where many one-offs can be found, she stood out.

And she was always thinking about other people. A few days before the funeral, I was sorting through Annmarie's purse and tucked away in one of the pockets was a piece of paper. Opening it up I saw it was pretty much a "bucket list" of things she wanted to do:

1. **Perfect health;**
2. **Winning millions on lottery;**
3. **My family's health and happiness;**
4. **Buying Rhiwlas;**
5. **Roddy going to Christ College;**
6. **Boys doing well in exams;**
7. **Going on fab summer hols;**
8. **My own housekeeper and driver;**
9. **Being loved and loving helping people with illness and the homeless;**
10. **Taking Ger to Bora Bora.**

Apart from the perfect health wish, which I don't think anyone would begrudge her, all her wishes would have allowed her to do something for other people. Being selfish, I particularly liked No.8, because her current housekeeper and driver was a particularly deserving case! No.10 was something we saw in a hotel magazine when we were staying in the Sofitel in Paris. It had pictures of all the hotels in the chain, and we were really taken by the one in Bora Bora. "One day..," she said. I will have to see how many we can still achieve for her.

I know I can't be objective about her so I asked one of my friends to jot down what he thought of her:

*My first impressions of Annmarie? Well I thought she was great – Merthyr is a town full of strong, confident women who have something to say (which isn't the same as talking a lot), and Annmarie is definitely one of those. She was certainly someone you'd pick out of a crowd – and that's a good thing, as far as I'm concerned. She sounded like a woman who didn't take any prisoners – which is fine by me because I don't take them either – and she appreciated the same quality in others. She was definitely someone who enjoyed a bit of banter, or a lot of banter if you were any good at it.*

*As I got to know her better, I realised that she may have had a tough exterior – you can't grow up in Merthyr and not have – but inside she was as soft as silk, and at the heart of her was the thing that mattered most: her family. Geraint and the boys, Pauline and her much-missed father Roy, sister Kath and her husband Steve and the twins, Avalon and her family, and then her closest friends. Annmarie was the ultimate people person – if she'd been on Twitter she'd have had thousands of followers because she could get on with people like nobody's business. You could see why she was a good businesswoman: she liked people and had the gift of the gab, which is a killer combination.*

*Our lives were so much better for her being in them, and are now so much poorer because she is no longer around to give you a nudge in the ribs and tell you not to be so pompous, or let loose on some poor acquaintance who was making too much of themselves, for no good reason. She was no respecter of others' phoney airs and graces – and no adopter of them either. The edge of her tongue, though often keen and well-aimed, was never malicious, which is a far rarer characteristic now when so many can be constantly carping and mean-spirited. And there was something else too: if Annmarie was giving you a hard time, she must have thought you were worth it. Woe betide those she left alone, for they were truly irredeemable.*

And as for my thoughts about Annmarie, well that's obvious. She was the boys' mother. Pauline's daughter. Kath's sister. Avalon's best friend. A rock for those who needed her, and a comfort too. The best company in the pub for friends when times were good. The shoulder you needed to cry on when times were hard and the world was a sad, small place. She was all this and more for them.

And for me? She was – is – my wife and my Princess, and I love her.

# And finally

*No one who knows Annmarie will be surprised that she would have the last word in this book: she did it in life, so why should this be any different? Going through her papers, Geraint found a handwritten note of sayings, quotations and maxims, which we subsequently discovered appears on Oprah Winfrey's web blogs. This seemed to encompass Annmarie's philosophy perfectly. It is reproduced here as found.*

**What do we know for sure?**
1. What you put out comes back all the time – no matter what.
2. You define your own script. Don't let others write your script for you.
3. Whatever someone did to you in the past has no power over the present. Only if you give it power.
4. When people show you who they are, believe them the first time.
5. Worrying is wasted time. Use the same energy for doing something about whatever worries you.
6. Whatever you believe has more power than what you dream or wish or hope for. You become what you believe.
7. If the only prayer you ever say is 'Thank you' then that will be enough.
8. The happiness you feel is in direct proportion to the love you give.
9. Failure is a signpost to turn you in another direction.
10. If you make a choice that goes against what

everyone else thinks, the world will not fall apart.

11. Trust your instincts. Intuition doesn't lie.

12. Love yourself and then learn to extend that love to others in every encounter.

13. Let passion drive your profession.

14. Love doesn't hurt. It feels really good.

15. Every day brings a chance to start over.

16. Doubt means "don't". Don't answer. Don't rush forward.

17. When you don't know what to do, get still. The answer will come.

18. Trouble don't last always.

19. This, too, shall pass.

20. I will act with the intent to be true to myself.